*1*

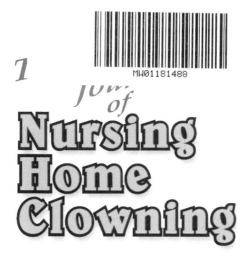

*Joy of*
# Nursing Home Clowning

*Author:* Anita Thies
*Illustrator:* Bill Moore
*Cover Design:* David Maser

*Contributors:*
Judy Barker
Karen Baxter
Brian Black
Karen Boudreaux
Bobbi Chard
Randy Christensen
Charlotte Cochran
Cathie Degen
Linda Forrest
Hal Grant
Julie Jahn

Carole Johnson
Carol Kay
Jan Kerr
Paul Kleinberger
Susan Kleinwachter
Aurora Krause
Luella Krieger
Jacki Kwan
Ruth Matteson
Jennifer Mellinger
Tammy Miller
Pam Moody

Bill Moore
Karen Oke
Curt and Diana Patty
Kathy Piatt
Elizabeth Plozner
Bud Salloum
Shobhana Schwebke
Donna Shuster
Dr. Richard Snowberg
Trudy Stryker
Korey Thompson
Janet Tucker

Copyright 2007©
by Lighthearted Press
761 Cornwall Rd.
State College, PA 16803
ISBN # 0-9701379-5-8

Library of Congress Control Number: 2007901498
All photos in this book used with permission.

# Dedications

I dedicate this book with thanks to God who lifted me out of depression and gave me new life; to my mother who lived with courage through all her nursing home days; and to my husband Jim and son Bill for all their love and laughter. — Anita Thies

To the glory of God and to Carol, my partner in life and ministry, who has upheld me in all that I have tried to do and has brought me great joy I dedicate my drawings. I also dedicate them to Brooke, a special joy maker. — Bill Moore

## Special Dedication

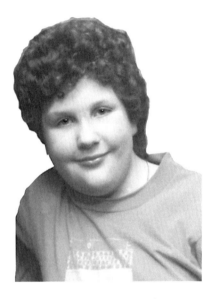

In Loving Memory of
Amanda Maser
1977-2005
Whose smile could light up a room
and whose heart for giving
knew no bounds.

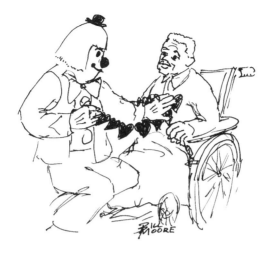

## Connecting Heart to Heart

In the presence of sadness
are you touched by compassion?
Do you long to bring laughter
where a smile never shines?

Do you see too many people
who don't know their own beauty?
Let them see it in your eyes
for without you they're blind.

So come be a dancer,
be a clown, be a mime,
be the friend of a puppet.

Come bring all the heart and the soul,
bring the love that God gave you to give away again.
Don't be afraid to be all that you are.
You're a gift to be given.
Enter in as a servant and stay as a friend.

© J W Rickert from the song "CMPD" on the
album "By Your Touch" www.jaimeRickert.com
excerpted with permission

# An Invitation

Imagine entering a family room where some three dozen clowns have gathered to meet you and share with you their passion in life.

They have come to tell you, in their own words, why they clown in nursing homes and assisted living facilities. They have come to share tips and creative ideas for your own clowning and guidelines if you're just starting out. They have come to encourage you with stories of their own journeys and of those who have touched their hearts.

I've gathered together some of the most experienced clowns I know to meet you in this book and have given them space to write about their experiences. I hope you'll see in the diversity of their experiences the many roles and opportunities that await you. For your gifts as clown and caring person are deeply needed.

I hope too that this book will provide you with a supportive community to cheer you on and that you'll feel a personal connection with all of us. I invite you to join in conversation with us using contact information in Chapter 13 and on our website.

I've included sections for specialized groups including "Junior Joeys," those who clown in Alzheimer's units, and those who are clowns in ministry. I hope the Santa Claus section will encourage you to add to your wardrobe and outreach.

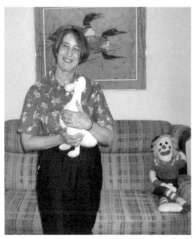

So I invite you to enter my "family" room, find yourself a comfortable chair and settle in. I'm so glad you're here.

*Anita "Toot" Thies*

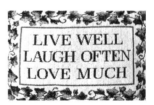

LIVE WELL
LAUGH OFTEN
LOVE MUCH

*My Mom's favorite pillow*

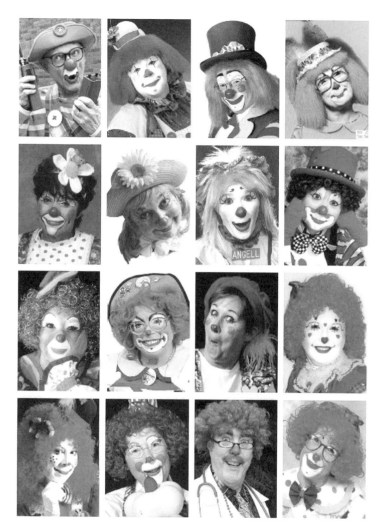

## The Clowns on the Cover (From left each row)

Top Row:        Dr. Richard Snowberg, page 54; Janet Tucker, page 70;
                Paul Kleinberger, pages 43 and 162; Julie Jahn, pages
                114 and 179.

Second Row:     Carole Johnson, pages 60 and 150; Shobhana Schwebke,
                page 28; Ruth Matteson, pages 152 and 156; Aurora
                Krause, page 91.

Third Row:      Judy Barker, page 76; Carol Kay, page 96; Susan
                Kleinwachter, page 86; Tammy Miller, pages 14 and 102.

Fourth Row:     Kathy Piatt, page 24; Donna Shuster, page 108; Rev. Bill
                Moore, pages 124 and 187; Anita Thies, page 186.

# Table of Contents

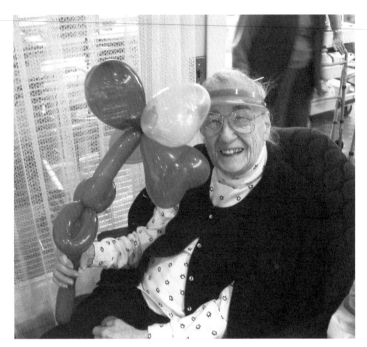

*Violet Weeden, 92, State College, PA*

# Chapter 1
# Is Nursing Home Clowning for You?

An aging woman once said she felt
like a "girl" with a grandmother's face.

> *If you'd like to see that face crinkle into a smile,*
> *perhaps nursing home clowning is for you.*

An elderly man once said he felt
like a "boy" yearning to play.

> *If you'd like to bring out that playfulness,*
> *perhaps nursing home clowning is for you.*

No other place offers you so many ways
to be a clown and to share yourself.

> *You can entertain residents in community rooms,*
> *in hallways or by bedsides, bringing laughter*
> *to their lips and a sparkle to their eyes.*

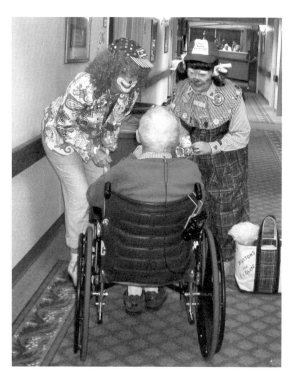

Connie "Freckles" Peters (left) and Linda "Buttons" Forrest visit with a resident at The Fairways at Brookline, State College, PA

With your caring clown visits,
you can be a special friend they long to see.

> *You can hold their hands and listen*
> *to their stories which are their truest treasures.*

You can seek to connect with those
whose eyes and thoughts seem far away.

> *You can join them in the moment*
> *and fill that moment with your care and presence.*

And in giving of yourself
you'll make an amazing discovery:

> *Without your ever seeking it,*
> *they will give you acceptance and appreciation.*

They will share their life with you
and give you the greatest of gifts:
their unconditional love!

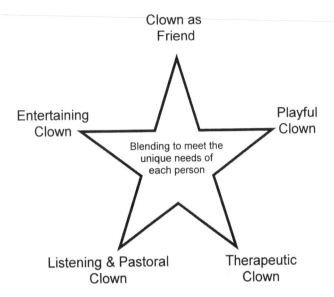

Clown as Friend

Entertaining Clown

Playful Clown

Blending to meet the unique needs of each person

Listening & Pastoral Clown

Therapeutic Clown

## Five Roles for a Nursing Home Clown

In coming chapters, a variety of clowns will share the emphases they bring to nursing homes. The diversity of their work reflects the many roles a clown may have in connecting with the needs of residents.

The star model for caring clowns* offers a framework for seeing these roles as "touch points" to meet the unique needs of each person you encounter. One role often leads to or blends with another, for instance listening is therapeutic and play develops friendship. The resident is always the "star" of your interaction.

These roles help address what some call the three "plagues" of the elderly: loneliness, boredom and helplessness. For the lonely, you can be a **Friend** and **Listener**. For the bored, you can bring stimulation and fun as **Entertainer** and **Playful Clown**. For those feeling helpless, you as a **Therapeutic Clown** can give them choices and bring to them the physical benefits of laughter.

In every case, your personal attention and sensitivity to them can lift their spirits and help their "star" to shine.

* *The star model was introduced in* The Joyful Journey of Hospital Clowning: Making a Difference with Love and Laughter © 2003 Lighthearted Press.

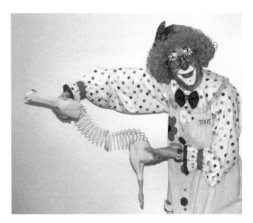

*Though we may
no longer be a
"spring chicken,"
we can put
a new "spring"
in our step
at any age
by exercising
our funny bone
and "stretching"
the realms
of possibility.*

## Chapter 2:  Humor for the Ages

One gift we bring to residents is that of humor and its transforming power. Humor can help change how we view a situation, how we view others, even how we view ourselves.

I'll always remember how U.S. President Ronald Reagan used humor after he was shot in 1981. He quipped to his wife, "Honey I forgot to duck," and told his surgeons, "I hope you're all Republicans." His use of humor showed mastery in a crisis situation and reassured the nation of his coping skills.

Every time we laugh with residents, we are emphasizing the value of humor. We are encouraging them to take themselves more lightly and to practice humor themselves.

A clown can also "empower" residents and bring forth their sense of wonder and play to enhance healing, says Ermyn King, who brings interactive drama, puppetry, dance/movement, storytelling, and integrated arts experiences to patients and families in her role as Arts Program Specialist at Children's National Medical Center in Washington, D.C.

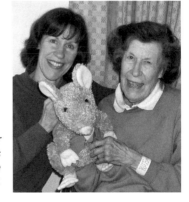

*Ermyn King is shown at right with her
mother, Jeanne King, after a clown's
visit to the rehabilitation center where
her mother was having a short stay.*

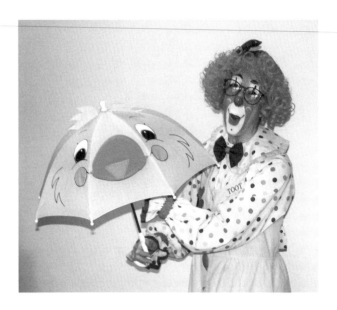

## When a Smile Is Your Umbrella

*Just let a smile be your umbrella*
*on a rainy, rainy day.*
*And if your sweetie cries just tell her*
*that a smile will always pay.*
—by Sammy Fain, Irving Kahal and Francis Wheeler

In my community room programs, I often play a recording of this song while residents clap and sing along. Most grew up with the song, written in 1927 and later recorded by Bing Crosby and Perry Como, among others.

While they sing, I twirl my smiling duck umbrella and hand a volunteer a long red balloon. Holding each end of the balloon in their hands, they can easily bend the balloon into a large upward curve for a smile and then turn it upside down and hold it over their head to represent an umbrella. I give other residents scarves to wave, signifying the "rain."

It's a peppy, upbeat song they enjoy enacting. But I've learned that it can be even more than that. I've seen that, for some, a smile and the courage to laugh in the face of adversity can become a powerful personal approach to living.

## The Courage to Laugh

I've seen that in Violet Weeden, one of the residents who has captured my heart. (Violet is shown below and on page 8.) I am grateful for her permission to share her story. Violet moved into assisted living nearly three years ago and is still sorting through things at her former house while also battling pancreatic cancer.

"I kept waking up in the middle of the night thinking I'm terminal and I don't have my house cleaned out," she says. "And then one night I realized that I'm not the only one who's terminal. Everybody's terminal. And I just laughed about it—right there in the middle of the night.

"And it was a turning point—I reinvented myself. I was reading today about the statistics of survival with my kind of cancer and I don't know really what I'm living on—I'm living on a smile. Laughing has been a protective thing—just to be able to look at things in lighthearted ways. You quip and just try to make others smile."

I asked her what makes her laugh and she said, "Thinking about going to the dentist."

How so? "Well I told my doctor I didn't want to spend more money going to get a cavity filled if I'm going to die right away and he said to me 'go to the dentist.'"

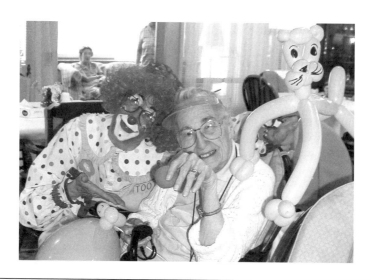

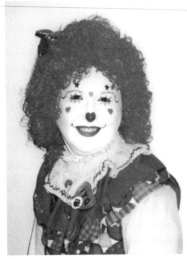
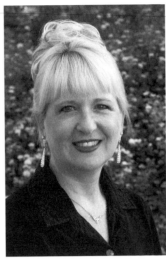

### Humor for the Ages:

## How Laughter Makes a Difference

#### By Tammy "Hugz" Miller

Many people might call me a "clown" even without the grease paint, but I do love to laugh and help others find the joy of laughter. My life of clowning has taken me to almost every venue a clown can enjoy— from large corporate events to one on one visits in hospitals or nursing homes. From my hometown to larger cities to international travel where I taught clowning and visited orphanages and hospitals in remote villages of Bulgaria, this world of clowning has been fun, exciting, and never dull!

### *Laughter Brings Us Together*

In Bulgaria, we interacted with people of all ages and, although we did not speak the same language, it was very clear that laughter is the same in all languages, and no matter what your age, laughter is a bond that brings people together!

Although today I do more professional speaking as a "plain clothes clown" talking about humor and healing than I do in full clown make-up, the value of humor for all ages is more apparent now than ever before. As our population is aging, there is more research being done on ways to keep our mental awareness sharp and functioning for longer periods of time. One of the ways that is being examined is through the use of humor. Humor is a way to help keep the mind sharp and in some cases to escape for a short time to a more pleasant place in our minds.

### The Medicine of "Heart-y" Laughter

The health benefits of laughter have long been proclaimed, but now there is new medical research to back up what many of us have known—laughter is good for you! Not only is it good for your soul, but it also helps you through difficult times and illnesses, and now it has been proven to be good for your heart!

The latest is from researchers at the University of Maryland, School of Medicine in Baltimore who have shown that laughter is linked to the healthy functioning of blood vessels. Laughter appears to cause the tissue that forms the inner lining of blood vessels, the endothelium, to dilate or expand in order to increase blood flow.

The study, which is the first to indicate that laughter may help prevent heart disease, found that people with heart disease were 40 percent less likely to laugh in a variety of situations compared to people of the same age without heart disease. This is just one piece of medical research that backs up the connection between humor and healing.

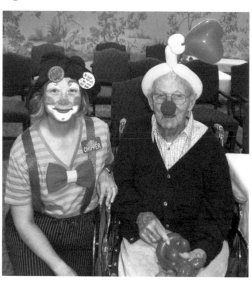

*Taking the adage of wearing your "heart on your sleeve" one step higher, Kenneth Walker joins in the fun with Sue "Chipper" Fetterman. New medical research shows that laughter is good for your heart.*

In the mid-1960's, Norman Cousins was diagnosed with a degenerative disease that left him in great pain and with no medical hope for relief. He checked himself out of the hospital and along with a high regimen of vitamin C he also took in a high dose of HUMOR!!! He watched his favorite comic routines (a BIG fan of the Three Stooges) and looked for reasons to laugh everywhere. At the very basics, he discovered that 20 minutes of laughter gave him two hours of pain-free time.

His fantastic healing was documented in his book *Anatomy of an Illness as Perceived by the Patient* (Norman Cousins, W.W. Norton & Co., 1979) which led to some of the earliest medical research into the humor and healing connection.

### Meeting the Unique Needs in Nursing Homes

Humor can benefit healing in many ways and through many methods. The nursing home setting has unique needs in that many people living in nursing homes are also battling loneliness and boredom. Whereas a hospital stay is generally considered temporary, life in a nursing home can be long term.

There are situations in the nursing home where you are helping someone deal with anger or frustration about being there. Some may miss their former home and not believe their stay here is necessary. As a clown walking into this setting, it is important to understand the great value you have for the residents with whom you interact.

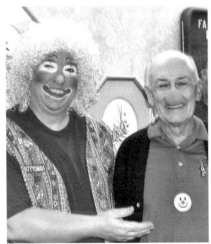

*Not only are residents looking for opportunities to laugh but so are family members.*

*Here Yvonne "Blooper" Mollica shares a smile with Truman Hershberger, husband of a resident at The Fairways at Brookline, State College, PA.*

*Mr. Hershberger shares special moments with his wife Dorothy by reading to her every day from the Bible. In her five years in the nursing home, he has read her the whole Bible twice and the New Testament three times.*

## *Spreading Giggles*

The sharing of the gifts and gags that you bring to the residents is not a small matter. As a clown you can engage your audience and leave something for later. Then that person can spread their giggle to the next person—maybe a caretaker or family member and so on and so on. This is one of the greatest aspects of what we do—laughter is contagious!!!

Just leading a round of good, strong belly laughing can encourage others to laugh along and clear out the "cob webs" and there is no cost for this activity. When I lead belly laughs, I try to throw my whole self into it. Be sure to laugh with gusto!

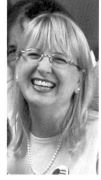

*Tammy Miller leads a hearty belly laugh.*

Clowning one on one is different than clowning on a stage or with a group. Some people shy away from this because they feel they have to be funny. Humor is found at all levels from the great big belly laugh to the warm, fuzzy feeling with a sweet smile and everything in between.

One of my favorite examples of various types of laughter is in the Disney film Mary Poppins. There is a great scene about all types of laughter. Just watching it you cannot help but laugh! This skit in itself can be funny and taken into a nursing home. You could provide examples of the laughter you see and ask the residents what type of laugh they have or the people they know have.

Around the world you hear of more laughter clubs starting than ever before. Humor leads to laughter which leads to healing at all ages. In the nursing home setting, the issue isn't always "healing" in the same sense that we relate to in the hospital, but an issue of providing an opportunity to laugh and feel better inside! The benefits of laughter are truly ageless and your role in bringing laughter, on a variety of levels, is a gift that is as rewarding for the resident and caregiver as it can be for you, the clown. The biggest step in doing nursing home clowning is the step through the door!

*Visit Tammy at* www.tammyspeaks.com *and see pages 102 and 195.*

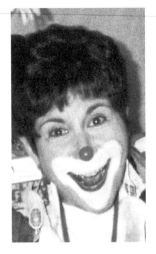

## Humor for the Ages:
# Making Positive Connections
### By Jacki Kwan, LCSW-C*

Humor is more involved than simply telling jokes or doing funny slapstick. Humor is being in a positive state of mind. People need different things at different times in order to be in "good humor." Some people need to laugh, while others simply need someone to sit and breathe with them.

I know from personal experience that even a nano-second of exposure to positive humor can make a difference. When you laugh or smile, you are in the moment when fear is absent, joy abounds and hope is reborn. I have seen this magic time and again with my own challenges in life as well as with the lives of those I have touched.

Humor, as it pertains to Humor Therapy, is never hurtful nor does it degrade a person's spirit. It's always uplifting. It gives people a temporary release of any negativity they are harboring.

### Allow People to Have Their Own Space

One of the greatest challenges for me is allowing people to have their own space when they really don't want to interact. I know in my head and in my actions that I give them that space they need, although it's difficult for me to accept the fact that some people would rather stay sour.

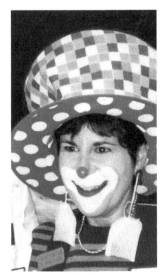

I realize, however, that those people are where they need to be emotionally. And for that I have the utmost respect.

*\* Licensed Certified Social Worker—Clinical*

### Listen with All Your Senses

As a result of my NLP training (*Neuro-Linguistic Programming*) and techniques I learned at Clown Camp®, I developed certain behaviors that help me connect with others.

You must "listen" with all of your senses: hear what the person is saying, i.e. *content* as well as *how* they speak. Is the other person's voice high or low? Soft or loud? Raspy or clear? Quick or slow?

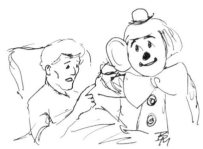

Next, see what the other person is doing, i.e. look at their facial expression; notice gestures and posture; pay attention to how you feel when you are with them. This may give you clues for how the other person is feeling.

### Ask Permission Before Touching

Since I am a psychotherapist, I am very aware of how many people do not want to be touched. It's kind of sad, actually. Anyway, I always ask people if they want a hug before I give one. I will offer my hand, and if they choose, they will take it. If not, I respect their wish.

Before I interact with someone I make sure that I have a referral, which can come from the patient/resident, from staff, or from a visitor/family member. Then the person still has the last word as to whether he or she is up for this kind of company. I particularly look for eye contact when I walk in the halls. If someone does not look at me, then I respect the other person's space and keep on going. I do not want to force the interaction.

I use the information I gather through my senses and try to mirror back as best I can what I sense in order to establish a connection. By practicing these rapport skills, I'm able to "see" with my ears, "hear" with my eyes, and "touch" with my heart.

*Excerpted with permission from* Almost Home: Embracing the Magical Connection Between Positive Humor & Spirituality (2002) © Jacki Kwan *Jacki has created HA!HA!LOGY® , a multi-faceted therapeutic humor program for health care facilities. See* www.hahalogy.com/ *and page 194.*

# Chapter 3
## Understanding Your Audience
By Jennifer Mellinger, C.T.R.S.*

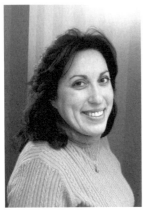

*Jennifer Mellinger*
*\* Certified Therapeutic*
*Recreation Specialist*

A clown visit is a change of scenery for our residents. It stimulates them to think of something other than their problems. In all our activities, we try to keep them "moving" through the day so they have something to occupy their time and are not thinking about their aches and pains.

Also if they are actively engaged during the day, they tend to sleep better at night. We try to bring in people who are new and different. Pet therapy groups stimulate them in a different way. And music—they love music and sing alongs.

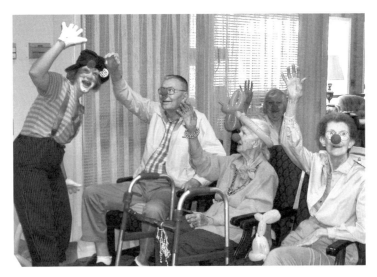

*Sue "Chipper" Fetterman clowns with (from left front) Bill Shoemaker, Ruth Toretti and Carolyn Aull and (at rear) Mary Lou Snitger at Brookline, State College, PA.*

## What Clowns Bring

Clowns bring them fun and make them laugh. This helps them to remember a lighter part of life. They say laughter is the best medicine and it's true. The clown visit is all very positive and positive breeds positive.

After a clown visits, we hear the residents talking about it. They say, "Did you see this?" It has stimulated them to remember, and this is continuation of the joy they received and often it continues for days afterwards.

The residents' minds are stimulated by familiar items. You need to connect with some part of them. The past is an easier place to reach because many have lost their short term memory.

Most were born in the early 1900's to the 1930's. Most of the men served in World War II.

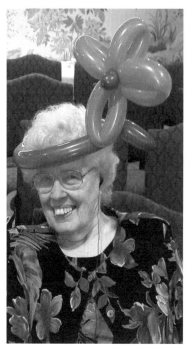

*Anita Thies met Norene Bigelow in a class on "Discovering Your Passion." Going strong at age 92, Norene brightens the lives of fellow residents through caring notes and smiles.*

### Creative Props Connect with Their Past

When you clown, consider using items that were part of their everyday lives to help stimulate their memories. For instance, use an old washboard in music. Or use spoons as an instrument or sand blocks or oatmeal boxes because they used them back in "the old days" when other instruments were not available.

Or use one of those hand-cranked hand mixers that makes noise, the kind they or their parents used. You don't need expensive props but you do need creative props.

The nursing home population requires a different level of communication. Your speech may need to be slower and you

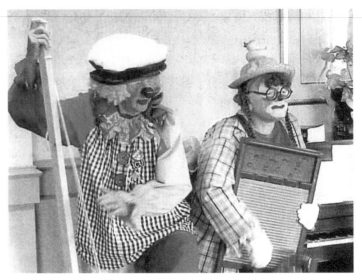

**Memorable Instruments**
*Peggy "Sunflower" Cole (left) plays a wash tub instrument while Dottie "Nancy Lou" Hummel strums a washboard. Such everyday items from years gone by help stimulate memories.*

need better enunciation so they can hear you more clearly. Your actions need to be more flamboyant so they catch your meaning. Color could play a big role in making you easier for them to see. Sometimes a smaller group is better for individualized attention.

You should also know that people with certain diseases avoid eye contact so that makes it tougher to connect.

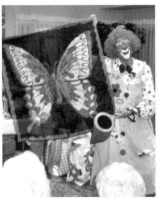

*Large, colorful silks help residents "see" your point.*

### Know the Home's Rules and Regulations

Volunteers who come on a regular basis need to meet all the home's protocols including signing confidentiality forms. You'll also need to comply with any state regulations. For instance, Pennsylvania requires a criminal background check. Also you should just know the home's basic procedures such as what to do if a fire alarm goes off so you can be of help.

## *Why I Love This Population*

People love going to see kids because they are at the beginning of their lives but sometimes people have a hard time accepting the end of life. Those of us who work in assisted living facilities and nursing homes don't see it as the "end" of life but a continuation of life. We can learn so much from this generation.

I love this population because they're very giving, very knowledgeable. They're unique.

Many times outsiders have misconceptions of the reality of aging. I've lost both my parents, but I feel I have 95 moms. They are just so giving. They care about you as a staff member as if you were their own children.

Once you get to know them as the people they are, you see past their limitations. Just because they can't walk as quickly or as easily as you doesn't mean they have less to give or are less appreciative or less fun. We have a heck of a good time.

*Jennifer Mellinger is the Activity and Volunteer Coordinator for Assisted and Independent Living at Brookline, 1930 Cliffside Dr., State College PA 16801*

*Feeling "tip-top," Nancy Thilo (left) and a fellow resident at Brookline join in the spirit of fun.*

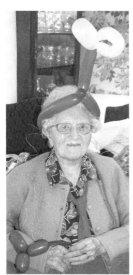 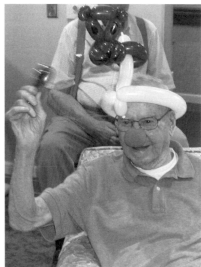

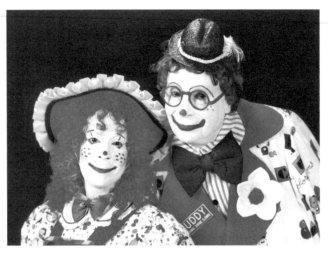

*Kathy "Popcorn" Piatt and her father Bud "Buddy" Salloum*

## The Wonder of a Wiggling Toe
### By Kathy "Popcorn" Piatt

I have enjoyed the joyful journey of clowning for almost 30 years, thanks to my father. Bud "Buddy" Salloum of Edmonton, Canada, starting clowning as a Shrine clown. He would come home from nursing home clowning telling me heart warming stories about the smiles he created and the new friends he made.

I remember my first nursing home visit with dad. I was eager to meet wonderful older people with great stories to tell.

Nothing prepared me for my first experience. I found many seniors with severe health problems, some with vacant stares and others hooked up to many machines. We went and visited some at their bedsides and others gathered in small groups. Some didn't even look up at us. I left that day in silent shock—not thinking I made one bit of difference to anyone or made their day any brighter. It all seemed so sad and depressing.

I agreed to go with my father to a nursing home again, not wanting to admit my fears or sadness. It's amazing, though, how wonderful life is when you shift your perspective.

This time I saw some beautiful elderly folks with eyes that danced. I saw smiles that I never noticed before. I talked with some who just wanted to chat. I realized then that we may never know if and how much joy we may have briefly shared.

### A Life-Changing Moment

My life-changing nursing home moment came when we went to visit a lady almost completely paralyzed with multiple sclerosis. All she could do was blink her eyes and on rare occasions wiggle her toe. The nurse told us after our first visit, her toe wiggled. On our next visit, the nurse said, "Look at her toe, she's happy you're here."

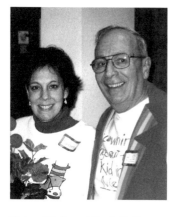

*Kathy Piatt and Bud Salloum*

That wonderful lady passed on more than 20 years ago but every night I wiggle my toe and say good night to her. Who's getting the rewards here? I thank my father and Our Father God for showing me how special and rewarding nursing home clowning can really be.     *To contact Kathy and Bud, see page 196.*

# Finding a Missing Smile
## By Bud "Buddy" Salloum

At my first Clown Camp®, we visited a nursing home. Anxious to show off a just-learned trick I approached a gentleman in a wheelchair. My tricks worked like they were supposed to, but I failed to get any response from the man—or the wheelchair.

I asked instructor Betty Cash for help. She approached and without a word started looking under and around the wheelchair, motioning for the man to lean forward so she could look behind his back. The man responded by saying, "What are you looking for?" Betty replied, "I know there's a smile here somewhere, and I'm going to find it."

The man said, "I can't smile because I lost my teeth."

At that point all of us broke into some real belly laughs that lasted into the giggle stage. This story goes to prove there's always a way, and it isn't always the brilliant tricks you've mastered.

---

# My Mother Loved to Laugh

### By Anita Thies

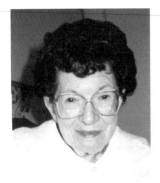

*My mom Ginnie Gosney*

Laughter was a hallmark of my mother, part of her Irish nature. She'd often begin a conversation with, "I heard this great joke..." Even if it wasn't great, she would laugh and so would those around her. One of her favorite songs was "When Irish Eyes are Smiling." Her eyes smiled a lot.

When she entered a nursing home, I learned ways to be a more caring clown and person. I learned not to judge on appearances.

My mom had a degenerative neurological disease called Progressive Supranuclear Palsy or PSP. Among other things, my mom lost the ability to talk, walk or move her eyes. But until the end, she was alert mentally. She just couldn't communicate.

I would see people who would talk to her as though she was mentally impaired, which she wasn't. I would see people not carrying on the energy of a conversation because she couldn't make eye contact. I would see people who basically "missed" connecting with her.

### Never Underestimate

And I would have too, had I not spent time with her and learned to read her in subtle ways. What I learned from my mom is never to underestimate the ability of residents to hear or to comprehend. With my mom, I became the keeper and voice of our shared memories. I carried the energy of the interaction. As a clown we often do that too.

In the last week of her life, when she lost the ability to swallow, I wheeled her out to the bingo game she always loved. She watched and listened as the staff played her card for her.

I learned from my mom the worth of living every moment right to the end. In clowning also, we need to stay in the moment, as hard as that may sometimes be to do.

*Excerpted with permission from the Hospital Clown Newsletter, Vol. 8, No. 2*

---

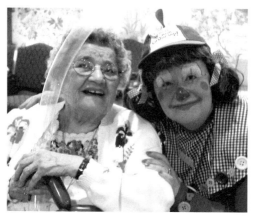
*Linda "Buttons" Forrest with Tess Martilotta*

## Different Than Hospital Clowning
### By Linda "Buttons" Forrest

I have enjoyed numerous hours of hospital as well as nursing home clowning. I have a passion for both, although they are very different from one another.

The patients in the hospital have a need to be humanized, i.e. treated as a person, not just a room number. Playing for a few minutes with a clown takes their mind from pain and worry. Most of these patients will get well and return to their homes.

Nursing home residents, however, are in a different stage of life where they will most likely not return to their own home. Some may have fond memories of the past, and have to deal with the loss of family and friends. Others may not remember the past but will be charmed by your smile and colorful clothing. Playing with a clown will make them forget their loneliness and make them feel special. Individual attention with a smile is healing!

Watching a clown show with other residents is a time for shared laughter and points of conversation after the clowns have departed. In both the hospital and nursing home settings, it is extremely important that a clown be a good listener and have a feel for each situation. Kindness and caring with a red nose and a smile will brighten a lonely soul and perhaps bring a smile to their face. *To contact Linda, see page 189.*

# Chapter 4

## Gifts from My Mis-Takes:
### *Developing the Quality of Our Caring Clowning*

By Shobhana
"Shobi Dobi"
Schwebke

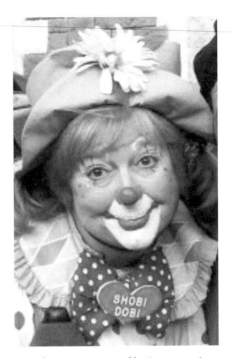

I want to share with you more of my process of being a caring clown than to give you advice. So many clowns come to me with the fear of making a mistake. Mistakes are gifts. In theater terms, a "take" is a little act. So this being said, I want to share with you some of my "*mis-takes*."

I tell you these not to discourage you, but because they made me do some deep reflections and gave me some important lessons in caring clowning. They also made me recognize my own fear of suffering and death and to clown to the healthy person and not the *dis-ease*. In total, they have made me a more spiritual person and a stronger person—a caring clown who does not run from suffering.

Once called "Old Age Homes," nursing homes today often have residents who can no longer take care of themselves at home and require full time care. That doesn't necessarily mean "old." I found this out on my very first outing. I visited many residents that day, but it is the *mis-takes* I really remember, because they were gifts in disguise.

The usual pattern at nursing homes, as I was to learn from experience, is for the staff to gather all the residents into a common room for the clown to entertain. I had been doing hospital clowning for a few years and was used to going from room to room. So when I finished my little meet and greet show, I asked, "Are there any residents here who can't leave their rooms?" The response came: "Oh yes, they're over in the East Wing." I asked, "Is it OK for me to go over and visit them?" "Oh they'd love it," the staff person answered, pointing me in the right direction.

With the confidence of a fairly seasoned hospital clown, I bounced over to the East Wing. It looked like a hospital corridor; however, there were no unit or charge nurses, no staff sitting around computers, no doctors walking around—nobody to ask whom I should see or not.

So I peeked into the first room and waved a greeting. "Would you like a visit?" I paused and posed and observed the room. The patient was a woman in her mid-twenties. There was classical music playing. The room had been well attended to with photos and flowers. I saw that the woman had some evidence of a muscular *dis-ease*. She seemed to take me in without a frown, so I tiptoed in with my usual cautious shy Shobi character.

Then I started to do a little magic show with my Mini Puppet. The woman's whole body began to jerk and she began to squeal. I had no idea if this was delight or horror. Was she happy to see me or terrified? Whom do I ask? What do I do?

### We Are Not Perfect

I went into the hall—still nobody around. I never did find a staff person to ask. In retrospect, after so many years of hospital clowning, I would have done the same thing. Did I learn something? Yes, I learned I was not to beat myself up if I didn't come up to my own expectations.

This is important in working in nursing homes. We are not perfect; sometimes we may be in the wrong place at the wrong time. Most of the time we have no idea of the ripples of joy we are spreading until someone tells us much later.

## The Magical Realm of Being in Character

I continued to clown on the East Wing and most of the rooms were no different from doing a hospital clown round. Then I came to a large room down the hall with three wide-awake elderly gentlemen all sitting up in bed. I waved at the door and they all smiled and one waved me to come in.

"Finally, I am going to be able to really clown with someone," I thought. So I bounced into the room. But to my utter surprise one of the men yelled really, really loudly, "Get the #*$%&$* out of here!" I reacted in clown character, jumping about a foot straight up in the air, because it really did surprise me! "Okey-dokey" I chirped, and hopped back out the door.

### Don't Take It Personally

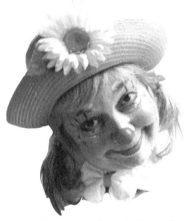

I stopped outside the room to recoup. After all it was really the first time Shobi had ever been yelled at. I expected my little girl clown to cry.

The interesting thing was I didn't feel affected at all. To my amazement, the angry words just bounced off. What I learned was that by keeping in character, I didn't take it personally.

This *mis-take* reinforced my belief in having a strong clown character. My personal ego was not involved in the incident. My clown character, Shobi Dobi, lives in a child wonder-filled life that is not affected by most of the adult confusing world.

Our characters can be a small quiet clown or a singing clown or a dancing clown, but all in the magical realm of being in character. As we all know "things go better in clown," and here I sensed a defense in being in a clown. It was almost like wearing armor or is it amour—love?

### Exquisite Caution

I'm not speaking about doing something irresponsible like going in really big and loud and giving someone a heart attack.

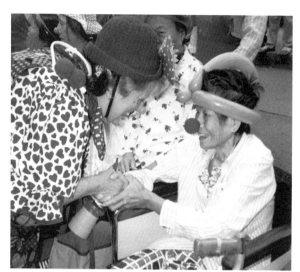

*During a trip to China, Shobi visits with a resident in a hospice facility.*

I went into that room with quiet caution. I call it "exquisite caution" because it is delicately pure in heart and intention.

### Our Spirit of Service

This *mis-take* got me thinking about selfless service—service without thought of reward. In my search for understanding, some months later I had the good fortune to take a weekend workshop with Frank Ostaseski, founder of the Zen Hospice in San Francisco. (You can read his complete article, Our Intention in Service, on my website www.hospitalclown.com)

### Paying Attention to Our Inner Appearance

Our spirit of service takes the same quality of mindfulness we pay to our outer clown. We pay attention to our costume, make-up and skills. As caring clowns, we need to pay the same attention to the development of our inner clown—the development of kindness, sensitivity, gentleness, compassion and non-attachment to rewards for service.

Developing a spirit of service for the caring clown is not a privilege, but a responsibility. There are many spiritual paths to the heart. We caring clowns share two. We are clowns and we work with those who are suffering. We perform and we serve. However, this sense of selfless service is what makes a caring clown different from a theater clown.

The caring clown develops a more selfless vision of clowning. We so often give up attachments to results of our performance, as a patient falls asleep in mid show, or any number of interruptions. We are there for the patient, not to show off a performance. We often never see the results of our actions until days or months later, if at all. By the nature of our job, we do not even expect results from our actions. This is selfless service.

### To Help or to Serve?

When we say, "How can I serve you," we offer what we have. It is not about status. It is about compassion. Egos are not involved here.

"How can I serve" is a different attitude than "How can I help?" This is not about helping a situation. We feel powerless when we can't help enough. To help means there is something wrong which needs fixing. That is a judgment. Too often when we help there is someone who is needy. We try to fill that need and we become needy also. To help is action often full of pride, self importance and a need for recognition.

Words are important in framing our attitudes. It is very important to replace the word "help" with "serve." In the beginning it is best to say it out loud in a whisper to yourself, as it is impossible to get more than one thought out of the mouth at one time (unlike the mind.)

Selfless service is an attitude which takes the vigilance of self-inquiry to master. It is important to watch how we offer our service. We need to be honest with ourselves and others about our intentions, and to know when we feel we need a reward and admit it. This seems obvious, but sometimes we want to do so much good that we overlook our real intention. It happens. It is human nature. However, if we don't recognize our feelings, resentment and bitterness can turn off the inspirational creative juices. It can lead to burnout and compassion fatigue. And it can close the heart—the very vehicle of the caring clown. It takes a mountain of our own good nature to lift us above complaints that can pollute the awareness of selfless service.

## Shobi's Practice

This is Shobi's practice. Before I walk into a situation—a room or a lobby—I take a deep breath, enter the room on the exhalation and take a clown pose. Exhaling on entry relaxes everyone in a room, on a stage, anywhere. Taking a big breath is what we do when we are frightened and excited. A big "ta tah" can work in the circus, but we are talking about a nursing home. When we exhale on entry or even walking up to a person, it is a relaxing gesture. This is quite the opposite of what most of us do by habit. Again, it takes some vigilance to change this habit.

During the clown pose I think *soft belly*, which relaxes my abdominal muscles. "*Soft belly*" is what Steven Levine uses in his hospice workshops. When I think *soft belly*, it pulls me out of my reactive mind and allows me to work out of my heart.

I make eye contact with the person(s) in the room. We've all heard it many times—eyes are the windows of the soul. For a caring clown it is most important to look beyond the body and into the soul, i.e., clown to the person inside not the *dis-ease*. So it has become my practice to not look at someone, but to look into their eyes.

As I survey the room, I ask myself, "How can I serve this situation?" I don't expect an answer in my mind; it is the attitude change that I am asking for. It clears my mind for intuition or one might say help from higher places. The answers come in my spontaneous clown reactions. Experienced caring clowns know we get a lot of help from higher places, and I am not referring to administration. You might think, "This will take too long," but remember again we are in a nursing home, not on stage. With repeated use, all of this practice becomes a habit.

When our mind is engaged in "How can I serve this situation," it leads to positive actions—not helplessness. It may mean getting out of the room or blowing bubbles, waving, holding a hand or giving a hug. Listen to the heart and allow a spontaneous response. The appropriateness that comes is always a surprise to me. I have learned to trust that higher connection.

## We See This During a Disaster

To serve is to give, to share what we have. This service is cooperation without judgment. We see this happening during a disaster—what is usually competition becomes cooperation. We support one another. Everyone pitches in to serve as best as they can regardless of title or rank. There is no place for pity and there is no status; everyone is equal. This is equanimity in service. When we are free from placing conditions on our work, it becomes selfless service. It is unconditional love and unconditional service. This kind of service is an act of love and a true act of compassion.

### Selfless Compassion

There is a companionship of mutual respect, dignity, wholeness and love in this compassion. This selfless compassion is what moves us into the spirit. Selfless service is mysteriously purifying. It continually replenishes our self-respect, as well as, respect for those around us. It puts us into the flow of the "divine."

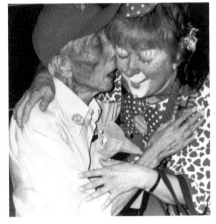

Selfless service allows a rich nectar to flow into my heart. It is grace in action. Inner knowledge sprouts from our hearts, creating rivers of love that can wash away fatigue and replenish the heart's compassion. Within the heart of the selfless server, love is boundless.

### Being Real – Know Thyself

Back on that East Wing with my "*mis-takes*," I entered a room with an intense odor. The man was having trouble speaking but beckoned me to come close. As he was whispering, I bent over him so I could hear him speak. There was a horrible smell coming from his body and I gagged. I was horrified at my reaction and did a little dance to try to turn to get back into character, but I was having trouble controlling that gag. Again, there was nobody in the room. He kept whispering so I got close enough to hear what he said: "Would you close the bathroom door?" I immediately did this, but that was not the cause of the odor. I found out later that it was from some sort of cancer. But at the time I was so embarrassed for not being able to control my gag. I thought, "Another failure to bring cheer to a room."

## We All Have Our Weaknesses

This weighed really heavy on my heart for a long time, making me do lots of research and again I learned many lessons. First of all, we all have our weaknesses. Some clowns will faint at the sight of blood. I don't. But I gag at vomit, body excrement and foul smells. I can't stop my gagging. Some clowns cannot be with a suffering child because they have a child; some of us see our own elderly parents in all suffering elderly patients. I don't have problems with human beings only animals. I can't stand to see a suffering animal.

We all have our ways. It is important to realize our own feelings. Only then can we overcome them or work around them. There is so much need in the world for a caring clown, so we can each find the right place that works for us.

## Resisting the Instinct to Flee

This *mis-take* was still on my mind. I wanted a more compassionate way of being in this situation. At the time I was reading *The Tibetan Book of Living and Dying* by Sogyal Rinpoche (Harper, San Francisco, 1992, page 316.) I came home and opened it up and read about this technique for arousing compassion for a person who is suffering: ". . . imagine one of your dearest friends, or someone you really love, in that person's place. Imagine your brother or daughter or parent or a best friend in the same kind of painful situation. What more would you want than to free them from their torment?"

So I learned to take advantage of the clown's performance freeze or pause, look into the patient's eyes and see my best friend. Mother Teresa described lepers she cared for as "Christ in all His distressing disguises."

### On a More Practical Level

Not being a saint, I sought out a more practical level, which I am not afraid to use. I now have a little spring skunk that lives in a bedpan on my cart. I also travel with a little skunk on a key chain. Pulling out "Flower" shifts the embarrassment of both patient and clown and shifts the focus to the play with the puppet. We can both laugh about human discomforts and the sometime horrors of *dis-ease*. And not the least unimportant: Humor can help the patient feel not so alone and isolated.

### On an Even More Practical Level

As I am in the habit of asking everyone for advice, one day I asked my dentist about this predicament. He said, "I keep a small bottle of orange extract nearby. When a patient has very bad breath, I just dab of it under his nose." So I also carry a little bottle of it in my pocket.

### The Gift of Presence

My very first *mis-take* was on one Christmas day. I was clowning in a room with a grandmother and her grandchildren, when I noticed a very elderly lady curled up in the next bed. I thought, "Oops!" So I pulled the curtain between the beds and sat down next to her.

I positioned my face where she could see me and I noticed a small hint of recognition. So I sat down next to her and not knowing what to do, I just watched her breath. This just seemed like the natural thing to do. She then began softly singing Christmas carols in some language I didn't recognize. I hummed along with her for a long while—tears flowing down across my makeup as her hand tightened around mine.

I had done something that I learned as an art therapist. That is to go to where the patient is. In this case I changed my whole attitude and sat down next to the patient because that is where she was. It is very important with elders and with persons with advance *dis-ease* to go to their comfort range. We many need to get very quiet, very small, and very slow. We may be able to coax them into a little game, a little smile or a little play. Then again we may not. But we need to go to their space, make eye contact, and listen with our eyes, ears, and hearts.

That was my very first day as a caring clown. I didn't know it then, but what I was doing was practicing conscious breath.

## The Magic of Conscious Breath

This is a technique which I learned at the Zen Hospice in San Francisco and I have been teaching it in all my workshops ever since. At first it was because all the nurses in my workshops would say, "Do you realize how important this is?"

Then I began to get such positive feedback emails. "My dad was dying and I taught all my relatives how to do the breathing and we took turns. My dad died so peacefully." Again and again I would get emails. So it not only works for caring clowns, but also for our friends and relatives.

Most people are very uncomfortable around those dying. It is our own fear of death we are facing. So when we are uncomfortable we get busy. Fix the flowers, fluff the pillow, talk of happy things, and on and on with the avoidance of death. All the while the dying long for our presence.

## Stillness is the Basis of Listening

This technique is so simple yet so powerful and it gives one a way to be still. Stillness is the basis of listening. If we can quiet ourselves, we can open up and listen not only to the person in front of us, but to any universal power that may influence our stillness. Attention to intention is also a very important caring practice and the basis for many healing practices. This exercise is designed for the care giver to give complete attention and loving intentions and therefore their presence to a patient.

If possible sit heart-to-heart, i.e., sit with your left side on the left side of the patient. Think *soft belly*, relax, and take a deep breath, allowing your breath to massage your belly. Allow the patient's hand to rest palm down on top of your palm. Gently support their hand. Now watch their chest as their breath goes in and out.  Match your breath to their breath so you are completely synchronized. You may need to slow down or speed up, depending on the patient. If their breath is stressed and uneven yours will be also, but you can slowly quiet the breath.

After some minutes take your right hand and gently place it over their forehead—a half an inch over the forehead so you are not touching the forehead. The patient will feel the energy and heat from your hand. During all this time you are matching the breath. After a while take your right hand and put it gently on top of the patient's hand, again keeping the breath matching. All this is done with the intention of opening up your heart and giving this person your love. Putting the hand over the forehead may be omitted especially if you are new at a facility.

It seems like such a simple thing, but breath is the very engine of our lives. There is a profound peace that comes from having someone sit with you like this, not only for the clown, but also for the patient. I always have everyone in my workshops try this as the care giver and patient. There is great comfort in having this stillness with someone. It is a profound companionship. After doing it over a period of time, sitting with a dying person becomes a great privilege.

I even taught this to the orphaned boys on a boat with Maria's Children in northern Russia. I thought we were going into a nursing home and I wanted the boys, ages 12-18, to be comfortable being with someone who is very old and frail.

As it turned out we went to a children's hospital. So much for communication! But I will never forget watching one young clown, Kolya, as he sat very quietly with a frightened 3-year-old just watching her breath. (See photo below) The child stuck to his side like glue the rest of the time we were there. He showed me that it is not just for dying or frail people, but young children also respond to this technique.

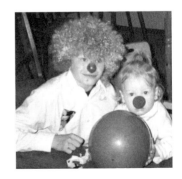

I have been told by other participants in my workshops that they even tried this technique with staff and family members who were upset. While listening to them, they would be aware of breathing with them. Then by slowly calming their own breath they would get them to slow down their breathing also, just standing next to them.

On a caring clown trip to Mexico I did a workshop at the beginning of the trip and taught this breathing exercise. Larry Jubal Davis of Selah, Washington, whose caring clown trip to Mexico was his first clown experience, recalls this experience:

"At a Guadalajara hospital, I approached an elderly woman. Her daughter was on her right-hand side. She was in quite a bit of stress. You could tell by the circumstances that her time was coming to an end. She was mumbling and her eyes were opening and closing. A nurse was on one side of the bed and her daughter on the other.

"I was at the foot of the bed and asked permission to hold her hand. I went around to the left side of the bed and picked up her hand and placed it on top of mine. I leaned over so she was able to see my face. Her daughter was telling her that I was a clown, but she did not respond in any way verbally.

"With her hand on mine, I placed my fingers on her wrist (pulse) and began to just look at her, took in her breath and watched her breathe. I watched her gestures and synchronized my breath with hers. As soon as I got my breath to synchronize with hers, she began to relax and after about two minutes of her relaxing, I placed my other hand over her forehead without touching it. I kept watching her breathe. Her eyes closed and she relaxed and started to breathe very freely.

"It kind of surprised me that this had really happened and I lost concentration on her breath so my breath became out of sync with hers. She immediately tensed up and started mumbling again. I concentrated again on synchronizing our breaths and she immediately relaxed. I removed my left hand from her forehead and placed it gently on top of her hand. It was amazing how she relaxed. Her daughter even relaxed. I stayed in breath with her for another few minutes. I then stroked the top of her hand and put it down. As I left her bedside, it seemed like her stress was relieved.

"What really happened was I connected with more than just with breath. It was like I was able to feel the stress and anxiety that was within her. I took some of that on into me, and when I entered into the hallway I was overwhelmed from the experience and had to get some assistance from some of the other clowns with hugs. I was able to deal with the experience. It was an experience that I will not forget."

### How Can I Clown Where There Is Suffering?

Another *mis-take* that made me ponder happened while visiting a nursing home at a Clowns International Festival in England. I passed the room of a man hooked up to several machines. His eyes were red and he looked so uncomfortable. My own empathy pained me right to the core. Was I supposed to go in and try to comfort this man? Did he even want me there? I felt the hurt so deep that it stopped me in my tracks. Was it my own fear of suffering? How can I transform this and clown? I never got to go into that room as the clowns with me pulled me off to a waiting bus. I did wave a little and smiled, but I didn't connect.

That look in that man's eyes stayed with me for a long time, so I wrote to several caring clown friends for advice and I took encouragement again from *The Tibetan Book of Living and Dying* by Sogyal Rinpoche who wrote, "If you suffer, you will know how it is when others suffer. And if you are in a position to help others, it is through your suffering that you will find the understanding and compassion to do so . . . So whatever you do, don't shut off your pain; accept your pain and remain vulnerable. However desperate you become, accept your pain as it is, because it is in fact trying to hand you a priceless gift: the chance of discovering, through spiritual practice, what lies behind sorrow."

Sogyal Rinpoche quotes Rumi: "Grief . . . can be the garden of compassion. If you keep your heart open through everything, your pain can become your greatest ally in your life's search for love and wisdom." [Rumi (1207-1273) was a 13th century Persian mystic and poet whose passionate poems of love and joy have been revered through the ages. UNESCO has declared 2007 as "Rumi Year."]

## Accepting the Place of Grief in Our Hearts

I realized it was not just my own fear of suffering, but the depth of the suffering I felt. It was a deep profound grief. I believe that is why grief has been given to us. It makes us live a little deeper in our

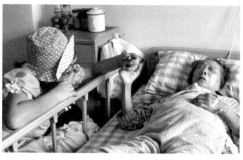

*Morighan Clinco visits with a man in hospice care on a trip to mainland China. She was 16-years old at the time and was Shobi's roommate for the trip.*

souls. We would not go that deep into our hearts on our own. But once we have accepted this deep place, and sit in its stillness, we realize it is lined with soft fragrant rose petals, and the view from that place is extraordinary.

So the next time I was in a situation with a profoundly suffering individual, I was a little more prepared. I looked right into the patient's eyes, and gave him the sweetest smile my Shobi could conjure up, and I sent him all the love through my eyes that I could. I was quiet; I was still, and I did nothing but stand there and breathe—breathe with him. Tears filled our eyes as they continued to meet. It was so sweet. He knew that I knew, and there was that moment of connection. He shook his head a little in affirmation. I gave him a homemade little angel for his bed table, "Someone to look after you." And I left. Later when I peeked into his room as I always do on the way out, he was quietly asleep.

### Stilling the Reactive Mind and Finding Inner Stillness

I have often said my *reason for being* is to glow. Clowning is a wonderful jewel though which to glow; however the clown is just the light bulb, not the source of energy. It is important that we are aware of allowing that light and lightness inside to shine through.

So often in a nursing home, we want to do something and we don't know what to do. So instead of being still, we get busy. We do a show, make a balloon, tell a silly joke and do anything but be still and make a connection.

We have all experienced how the mind can instantly say, "What if that is me in 30 years!" "What if that were my child?" The mind is a genius at multitasking. It can clown and think of many things at once. This is a "knee-jerk reaction." When the reactive mind kicks in, it boomerangs and strikes back at us with fear and it shifts our focus off those we are clowning for and onto ourselves.

I have a very active mind—much like my little dog—always curious, always going in many directions at once. If I get angry at my reactive mind, it just gets more active. Sometimes I gently visualize my mind as this little dog and pat it on the head with love, but more often I sit quietly watching my breath and the energy in my body softening my belly. This quiets the mental noise and allows me to be aware of the wonderful miracle of human existence. This is my practice. We all develop our ways of connecting through the doorways of our bodies. Every religion has its path to that stillness.

### The World on the Other Side of Our Senses

I visualize my being like a great ocean. So much can be happening on the surface, but beneath it is a still vibrant calm. Nothing that goes on can change that stillness as anything that reaches that depth becomes part of the vibrant calm. It is this vibrant calm that I bring into my caring clowning. The stillness flows outwardly as gentleness. Inner stillness and gentleness is beautiful presence in a caring clown; it spreads compassion in all directions.

♥ ♥ ♥ ♥ ♥

There are many articles free to download on my website www.hospitalclown.com. I don't consider them mine. They come from the universe in what I've begun to call the "hole in my mind." So I don't feel I own any of it.

I am just a clown vehicle and as I always say, "My clown car is fueled by love, gives off joy for exhaust, and drives on a highway of compassion."

How much better can life get? Well, maybe flying! And I know there are plenty of caring clown angels already doing that!

*To contact Shobi, see page 197.*

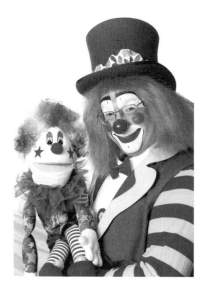 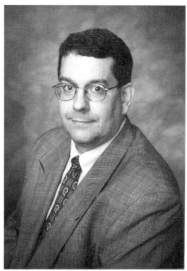

# Chapter 5
# Getting Started in Caring Clowning

By Paul "Fuddi-Duddy" Kleinberger

I have been a caring clown performing in nursing homes and extended care facilities on and off for many years. While it can be a very rewarding performing experience, and a great place to start for an aspiring caring clown, there are some unique challenges. For me, it was a learning experience just getting started.

I live just outside of Albany, New York. There are lots of clowns in my home area, as well as several clown alleys, troupes and groups. About 10 years ago, one alley I am active in decided it wanted to perform in nursing homes. We thought it would be a great way to fulfill our alley mission—to serve the community in a humorous way. At the same time, caring clowning was just getting its start in our alley. Several people interested in this aspect of the clown arts were looking for performance venues to practically apply what they were learning.

A committee of four members with caring clown perspective was assembled to explore the possibilities. My wife, Miriam (a.k.a. Senorita Soto) and I were asked to be part of the committee.

## A Performing Troupe of Caring Clowns

Our charge:  If feasible, put together a performing troupe of caring clowns to perform in area nursing homes.

Sounded simple enough!

At our first meeting, we determined that none of us knew anything on the subject. While we had all been performing clowns, and some of us had unique hospital experiences, we were all new to caring clowning and none of us clowns had yet to be inside a nursing home. We did not know anyone who worked at a nursing home, or so we thought. None of us had an idea on how to assemble a troupe of performers for such an effort. We had no idea how to build a program.

We had accepted the challenge only to quickly learn that we were a bunch of zeros! Were we in for an education!

But we had two things to our credit:  1. We all had the sharing, caring heart of a clown;  2. We had a desire to succeed.

At our second meeting, we evaluated our resources. The mother of one of our alley officers was a resident in a nursing home a few blocks from where we conducted our alley meetings. We also learned that another alley in the area visited nursing homes from time to time. Its' efforts were headed up by a well known clown we all respected. We divided up our resources. A few of us would contact the nursing home, and a few of us would talk to the coordinator of the other alley's performance troupe.

I worked as a salesman at the time. It was pretty easy to adjust my daily routine. It fell to me to make an initial visit to the nursing home. As I was planning to do so, it dawned on me! One of my younger brothers had worked in a nursing home while he was in college. My Dad reminded me I also had a cousin who, as a registered nurse, managed a nursing home in southern New York State. I called both. I explained to each what we were up to, what we hoped to accomplish and I asked for help, any help.

My brother explained that it was the Activities Director at the facility where he had worked who made arrangements to present live entertainment to the residents. While he had never seen a clown perform at his facility, he had seen the performances of magicians, puppeteers, singers and choirs, both children and adults, as well as other performers. The residents always loved the visits, the performances and the attention. He suspected that if nursing home residents were up for it, they would love the color, energy and the performances of clowns.

My cousin told me she loved the idea and suggested I talk with the Community Outreach Coordinator of the local facility. She suggested I make an appointment, not just drop in. She further explained the categories of care given to residents including custodial care, physician monitored care, and extended skilled nursing care. She explained that not all facilities have the same type of residents and that the age ranges and alertness of residents vary significantly. The last thing she suggested was that we talk with the professional staff of several nursing homes to get a mixed flavor of responses. She concluded by inviting us, as "Senorita Soto" and "Fuddi-Duddy," to visit her facility. She said we could get a first hand visitation and performance experience under her guidance and oversight.

While we weren't able to make the trip to my cousin's facility, I did call the nursing home down the street and requested an appointment with the Activities Director. We contacted the other committee members and passed along my cousin's suggestions.

As a committee, we visited four or five nursing homes over the next couple of weeks. Each of us received warm welcomes, lots of information and invitations that reflected my cousin's invitation

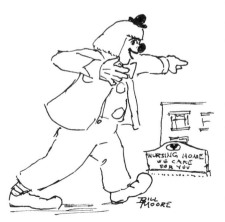

to climb into costume and make-up and come for a visit!

## When to Visit

What did we learn from the activities directors, nursing staff and the other professional staff members we met?

Performing clowns would certainly be welcome!

While many performers wanted to visit on weekends, it would be great if we could visit during the weekdays, in the early afternoons after lunch or the early evenings after supper. It would add variety to the normal day for residents as well as for staff.

### How Long to Perform

A "show" should be about 30 minutes long, probably no more than 45 minutes in length. Why? Many residents have short attention spans. Others have routines and schedules that must be maintained, depending upon the time and day of the week.

### Perform "with" the Residents

Audience participation during our performances was a must. Performing **with** residents was more important to the professionals we spoke with than performing **for** residents. The stimulation and interaction were considered very therapeutic and beneficial. Having fun and making our visits fun for the residents, their family and the staff was emphasized.

### Incorporate Singing

Singing should somehow be incorporated in to the program, if at all possible. Residents, especially seniors, love to sing and a group sing would be considered a big plus. The response to music, any music, was always positive.

### The More Laughter, the Better

We needed to make sure that laughter was the result of our efforts. The more laughter, the better. While the therapeutic aspects of laughter are truly appreciated, the general expectation is that clowns are funny. Nursing home residents have high expectations, justified or not, of performers who visit. The residents, as a group, can be quite critical. If they were disappointed, they had no qualms about expressing their disappointment. We should be prepared for such reactions. While "boos" were rare, they weren't unheard of.

### Include Visits to Rooms

We should include time to visit some of the residents who wouldn't be able to make it to the performance. Those who were bed bound, confined to their room for other reasons, or just unable to make it to the community room or cafeteria where we would perform would love to be visited, if only for a short while.

### Guidelines on Balloons

While we could certainly make balloons if we wanted to, what was most important was our willingness just to spend time with the residents. When it came to balloon making, we needed to be aware that some residents had allergies that balloons could aggravate. The nursing staff would make sure we knew who not to present balloons to.

### Stickers Are Good

Face and hand painting were probably not a good idea, except on family visitation days or holidays when children were prevalent in the facility. Stickers, however, were a great idea.

### Be Understanding of Families

In some cases, family members could be quite demanding. We should recognize the importance of their visits and be both flexible and understanding during our visits and performances.

We should be ready for anything.

Additionally, there were some general visiting guidelines we should be aware of that included the following areas.

### Touch with Care

Whenever you visit, always be supportive, affectionate and caring. Personal contact with others is extremely important for the residents.  Many times the only touch that older adults living in such a facility experience is when they are dressed or bathed.

Residents in nursing homes need to know they are loved and not forgotten. If they are receptive, hold their hand for a moment or two after greeting them. If you are a hugger, and many clowns are, give them hugs when you arrive and leave. Be sure to make eye contact when they are talking to you and you to them. Eye contact is very important.

### Schedule Visits in Advance

Plan your visits in advance with the staff. While dropping in at some facilities would certainly be okay, it is best to call ahead and make arrangements for a visit and a performance.

It is important for residents to retain as much control over their lives as possible. Knowing that you are going to be visiting and performing and being allowed to decide if they are going to participate with you gives the residents the opportunity to have some individual control over at least part of their daily schedule.

## Three Parts to Your Visit

As a performer, you must remember that, for the residents, there are three parts to a visit by a clown troupe:

- The residents looking forward to your visit and performance;
- The visit and performance itself;
- And the residents talking about it with everyone afterwards.

Planning your visits ahead of time allows for all three to happen.

### Provide Advance Pictures

Be sure to provide promotional materials, posters and group photos, if at all possible. Planning ahead allows the residents the enjoyment of anticipating your visit and performance. It creates a healthy buzz within the residence.

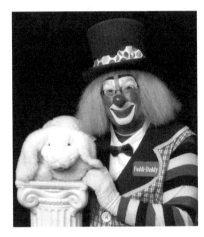

### Listen Attentively

When interacting with the residents, listen attentively to them and on an individual basis. Do not dominate the conversation or talk "at" them. Being a good listener allows the residents to talk about and enjoy their memories, as well as their current thoughts by sharing them with you while you are visiting.

Be sure to speak to all the residents as the adults, the teens or the children that they are. Do not be surprised that some of the adults you may meet may seem quite child like.

### Always Be Respectful

Always be respectful. Keep in mind that treating older adults like children, even if they are frail or cognitively impaired, does not foster their self-esteem. Failure to show the proper respect could cause resentment. It bears repeating: Always be respectful and use the traditional titles of Mr., Mrs. and Miss when you know their proper name. Use Sir or Ma'am if you don't.

### Share News and Funny Stories

When you visit, share news about what is going on in the outside community with the residents you meet. Feel free to talk about your clown and share stories about your troupe, where you have been, what you have done, where you are going next, etc. And don't forget to bring photos to share and leave with the residents. Be sure to share funny stories. Tell a few jokes. Even though residents are presented to you as a group, do your best to treat each one as an individual.

### Include Junior Joeys

Include Junior Joeys in your visits, if possible. Such visits for the Juniors can help make them aware of the aging process and help them understand that older persons need love and affection. At the same time, the senior residents typically enjoy interacting with youngsters. We learned that Junior Joeys in costume are always a hit. (For guidelines for Junior Joeys, see pages 156-161.)

### Be Friendly

Be friendly! While you are visiting, make it a point to say "hello" to all the residents you meet. There may be some who do not receive too many visitors. Interacting with all the residents you meet who live in the facility brightens everyone's day and it gives them something to talk about later.

### Remember the Staff

Do not forget the staff! Be sure to interact with the facility's staff members, professional, technical and support, and include them in your performances if at all possible. Be quick to thank the staff members and compliment them on their support of you and your efforts and what they do for the residents and their families.

## Therapy Animals

Therapy animals, while not popular when we were starting out, were not unheard of. While family pets were sometimes allowed to visit, a certified therapy animal would certainly be welcomed. Just make arrangements with the professional staff ahead of time.

## What NOT to Do

We also were advised of some things to avoid while visiting and performing in a nursing home:

- Never visit if you have a cold or another communicable ailment.
- Never enter a resident's room without asking permission to do so.
- Never open an outside door for a resident, even if they are insistent.
- When visiting in a resident's room, do not give a resident items that they could harm themselves with, especially things that are obviously out of reach.
- Do not remove any body restraints you may see.
- Leave the lifting and adjusting of resident's positions to the professional staff.
- Do not give any food to a resident without first checking with a nurse.

## Selecting Music

As we absorbed this information, we next looked at the singing. Several alley members involved in community and church choirs and one or two who were accomplished soloists suggested we start with audience participation type songs that were well known and easily sung.

Suggested were: "Row, Row, Row Your Boat," "In The Good Old Summer Time," "A Bicycle Built For Two," "Take Me Out To The Ball Game," and "New York, New York."

Getting the sheet music was a challenge, but, with the help of the Internet, we prevailed. And we learned during our first performance that it was true—the audience loved to sing!

The louder, the better! Plus, those types of rounds gave us the opportunity to perform simple clown antics that could start the audience laughing and clapping. Eventually, it proved to be a great lead in to our opening skit.

### Choosing Skits

Our committee members learned from the other alley visiting nursing homes that classic clown skits that were short and funny always seemed to be a hit with their audiences. So we initially built a show with skits we all were familiar with that didn't demand too many props, too much memorization or too much talent for that matter.  We included individual performances and routines as our clowns were moved and inspired.

We pulled together a variety of skits for single clowns, two clowns and groups.  These included clown classics like 3 plus 3, Ring Ring, Stage Coach, Taking My Case To Court, Wrong Number, The Painting, Peanuts, Mind Reader, Growing Taller and others. (See Skit Chapter pages 162-173.)

Then we asked for volunteers to get involved with us, the committee of four which had grown to six. At the time our alley membership hovered around 40 members, 25 of whom regularly came to meetings and public events. Our call for volunteers yielded another half dozen clowns, some very experienced and others new to clowning. We were surprised—we expected more.

We rehearsed one night a week for several weeks and as we did, a few more members joined us. When we declared ourselves ready for our first performance, we had 15 clowns ready to go, a dozen classic clown skits and routines, and music we thought would be fun and engaging.

### Having a Master of Ceremonies

A senior alley member took the helm of coordination. He contacted nursing homes, lined up performance dates and acted as our Master of Ceremonies as we presented ourselves and our performances. One of the first things we learned was that when he wasn't available, things quickly seemed to lose their continuity. Thus, we "auditioned" two more clowns to serve as our Master of Ceremonies so we would always have at least one back up.

## A Wonderful Time

Our first performance was wonderful. It was in a local facility and the residents proved to be very lively and interactive. They all joined in on the songs. They sang. They clapped. They laughed. They had a great time singing.

As we started in to our routines and our skits, they laughed and clapped some more and were truly appreciative of our efforts. When we reached out to include various staff members in what we were doing, the residents loved it. As I recall, it all went according to plan. We had a truly enjoyable experience.

The residents also had an enjoyable time and their continuing applause bolstered our self confidence. When our performance was concluded, we helped the staff wheel the residents from the cafeteria where we were performing back to their rooms. More than one resident yelled in to the rooms they were passing, "Look at what is pushing me down the hallway!"

After our performance, we visited several other residents. Balloons were made, stickers passed out, one on one routines performed and a splendid time was had by everyone.

During the next six months, we continued to get together weekly to rehearse, consider new material, and revise our program. We critiqued ourselves, tweaked our performances and looked for a skit that we could use to involve several audience members at the same time.

### Two Pivotal Happenings

Two things happened: A Northeast Clown Convention and "The King With A Terrible Temper."

Clown conventions certainly were not new to our alley. Several members, including Miriam and me, attended conventions on a regular basis. We often competed and made a good showing. What happened during this particular convention was that some of our nursing home performers entered single and group skit competitions and placed in the top three in both categories. When they told other alley members that their success was a direct result of participating in the nursing home troupe, more alley members got involved with us. This has become something of a tradition.

Alley members who intend to compete at clown conventions are welcomed in to our nursing home troupe and encouraged to polish their material and routines.

There are several versions of "The King With A Terrible Temper." (See it on pages 162-164) It is a funny skit that allows performers to go into the audience to find people to play the various characters in the story: The King, his three Daughters, a handsome Prince and, of course, a Fiery Steed.

It has proven to be a favorite. It allows troupe members to interact with the audience in a manner that other skits do not necessarily allow for. It is a routine that truly allows our clowns to perform "**with**" the audience instead of "for" the audience. It is also great for picture taking and memory making.

When we contact facilities for return engagements, the staff almost always asks, "You are going to do The King With The Terrible Temper, aren't you?"

### *An Expanded Outreach*

Our efforts have expanded over the years. Our nursing home troupe became our caring clown troupe. While we still visit many nursing homes, we also visit and perform in extended care facilities, memory care facilities, senior centers, senior day care programs, foster care programs, orphanages, and even the local Veterans Administration hospital.

In 2002, our caring clown troupe hosted some 40 clowns who were interested in learning more about caring clowning during the Clowns of America International Convention in Saratoga Springs, NY. After a session with our troupe, they were loaded onto buses and taken to a local senior center. They got a first hand visitation and performing experience. That visit in Saratoga Springs has lead to the formation of almost 20 similar troupes in clown alleys around North America.

*Paul Kleinberger is president of Clowns of America International, (www.coai.org) and a founder of Red Nose Response Inc., a charitable organization that brings love and laughter to those impacted by a catastrophe.(www.rednoseresponse.org) See the Skits Chapter by Paul starting on page 162. To contact Paul, see page 192.*

# Chapter 6: Clowning in Nursing Homes

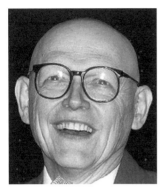

## How Are You?
## How Do You Feel Today?

### By Dr. Richard "Snowflake" Snowberg

Oh my, are there a lot of ways to react to these questions. In our society, when seeing someone we know, and even perhaps when introduced to someone new to us, we habitually say, "How are you?" or "How do you do?" or "How ya doin?"

This really is a cultural response, and one that is not necessarily followed in other cultures. In some Asian cultures, people exchange a greeting with a question as to whether they have eaten, and/or if they are hungry. This seems very strange to us, but then those not using our greeting might also think it strange that we are asking about someone's health—even if we have just been introduced to them.

The fact is that our greeting is hardly ever responded to in a truthful manner. Most of us say, "Fine, how are you?"

### How to Break the Pattern

When it comes to clowns, we can break the pattern of always asking after someone's health. If a non-clown sees me in my character, and asks, "How are you today?" I respond by saying:

### "If I was any better, I'd be twins!"

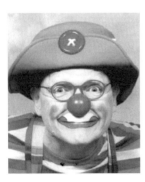

By doing this I break the cycle we usually parrot, and also create an amusing response that nearly always gets both a laugh and a smile.

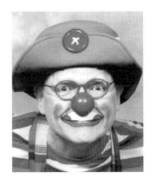

### *"I Have New Socks!"*

If I am the first to address someone verbally, I might say something very inane such as, "I have new socks!"

This type of response is so unusual it normally gets a similarly fun reaction.

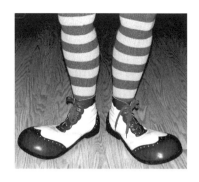

### To "Entertain" Means "To Focus Attention"

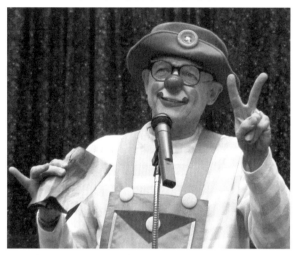

As caring clowns making rounds in nursing homes, it is important to remember you are there to entertain. As I've stated perhaps hundreds of times through some of my other writing, the word "entertain" means "to focus attention." We should strive to focus residents' attention on something besides themselves or their physical condition. Notice how I'm getting back to the introductory questions?

### Different from Hospital Clowning

Caring clowns most commonly work in hospitals and in nursing homes. A distinct difference between these two environments is the reality that most nursing home residents are not going to improve, get better, or generally feel "fine."

(I recognize that we do have nursing homes serving as transitional sites for some recently released hospital patients that are not ready for a return to home, as they still need some daily treatments or therapy. These residents are a minority of those that clown visitors will be seeing in a local nursing home facility.)

So, it is my opinion that when clowning in a nursing home, we need to strive to focus our attention on all things not related to an individual's general health.

### Relating to Their Situation

When we, as persons with reasonably normal health, don't feel in *tip-top* condition, we show symptoms similar to many nursing home residents. We may be moody, not want to move around much, find food distasteful, and generally look at the world or our personal situation in a less than positive manner.

### Get Them "Outside" of Themselves

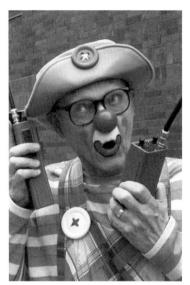

As clown entertainers, we should strive to get the residents *outside* of themselves. By this I mean, we should attempt to entertain them in such a manner that they forget about their personal pain and/or problems, and focus on that which you present or represent.

What is it that you can do to bring this about?

### Tap into Your Unique Experiences

Each of us has interests, skills or experiences which are unique. Use your skills or experiences to entertain your audience. A magical clown might carry around an arrow (Dizzy Arrow/Which Way Is Up?) and use a storyline about

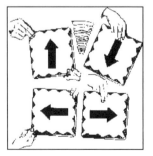

not being able to find his/her way around this home. Every time the performer turns the arrow card over to the backside, the arrow is pointing in a different direction. The performer scratches his head and explains that he/she keeps getting lost because the directional arrows keep changing.

### *Talk with a Puppet*

An entertainer utilizing a puppet might use that figure to carry on a conversation about the nursing home. One might even use the above mentioned problem of getting lost in the home, and have the puppet try to advise the clown performer how to get to the nurse's station, the dining

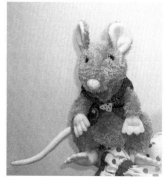

room, or some other area in the facility. The use of a puppet for purposes of carrying on a conversation means that the resident is not obligated to enter into a conversation with the performer. He or she can do so, but it is not necessary.

### *Draw from Your Hobbies*

If your performance skill is in fire eating or some other non-appropriate skill that is not useful or safe in a nursing home, take another approach to entertaining. Are you a good listener? Do you have hobbies from which you can develop materials for your nursing home visits?

Some clowns are stamp collectors or even scrapbook enthusiasts that do a lot of creative scrapbook layout pages with rubber stamps, craft paper, scissors and other tools. The latter might create some amusing scrapbook layouts featuring pets, famous people, the circus or perhaps children. All of these can be wonderful pages of illustrations to share with nursing home residents.

All of them can kindle memories and start stories that residents will recall for you. When the performer can get the audience in a nursing home talking more than the entertainer, they have created a very positive encounter.

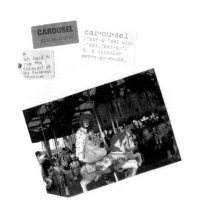

## Let Them Choose

While there are other techniques and ideas yet to be covered, it is a good time to consider what the above-mentioned scenario achieves. Caring clowns should always attempt to provide opportunities for their audience to make choices and decisions. Many times residents in nursing homes feel that they can no longer make any decisions in their life, no longer can give anything to someone else, or have any personal self worth. Anytime the performer can provide opportunities or actions that can counter these feelings or realities, success will be achieved.

The performer, in sharing scrapbook pages of clowns, pets, or travel illustrations, can ask their audience—the nursing home resident—which pages they'd like to see. By so doing, you have provided an opportunity for *choice*.

It seems a simple thing, but, to a nursing home resident, choices are sometimes few and far between. The resident will likely chose something of which they have interest. This being the case, the sharing of the selected topical pages will often elicit memories and conversation from the resident.

### Personal Entertainment in the Moment

Here the resident is using their rich and long history of personal memories to add to the performer's presentation. At this point the resident is no longer thinking about how they feel but is *in the moment* with the performer. Entertainment is taking place. And, the entertainment is personal as the resident has structured the experience to their liking.

If you are a balloon sculpturer or character artist, provide opportunities for choices, as to what creations will be made. If your skill is in storytelling, look around the resident's room and note any photographs, unique furniture, artwork or gifts that are

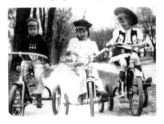 present. Then start to weave a story or, if the resident is receptive to conversation, ask about that which you see. In almost all cases, the furnishings and photographs found in residents' rooms all carry special meaning.

## If You Are a Newer Caring Clown

Newer caring clowns may feel at a loss due to the fact that they don't recognize the skills that they actually do possess. If this is the case with you, ask some other clown friends for their ideas as to what you can do for nursing home entertainment. If you ask people that you know, they can frequently flesh out ideas that you may overlook.

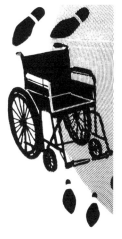

### 7 Starter Ideas

1. Do you have instrumental musical abilities?

2. Have you given thought to wheelchair dancing, sing-alongs, or wheelchair races?

3. Assist with snack deliveries to individual rooms; work along side other food servers in the dining room or cafeteria.

4. Volunteer to be the guest clown-number caller for bingo.

5. Help with delivery of mail.

6. Become a room inspector, checking for bunnies under beds.

7. Be a fashion police inspector, giving tickets to nurses and other health providers for inappropriate apparel, makeup or footwear.

| B | I | N | G | O |
|---|---|---|---|---|
| 23 | 3 Feather Dusters | 1 Clown Nose | 20 | 12 |
| 17 | 22 | 9 | 7 Happy Memories | 13 |
| 24 Smiling Faces | 16 | FREE BINGO SPACE | 10 | 2 Clown Shoes |
| 14 | 5 Finger Puppets | 19 | 8 | 15 |
| 6 Balloon Animals | 21 | 11 | 4 Kazoos | 18 |

Are you beginning to get the picture that there are hundreds of ways in which a clown can introduce himself/herself in a nursing home environment and not have to ask the question, "*How are you doing?*"

*Dr. Richard Snowberg is founder and director of Clown Camp ®, University of Wisconsin-LaCrosse* uwlax.edu/clowncamp/ *To contact him, see page 198.*

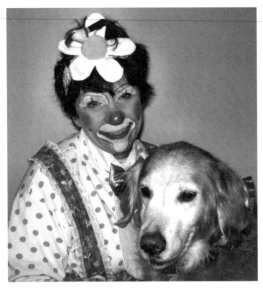

*Carole "Pookie" Johnson with her dog Gracie*

## Finding Your Niche

By Carole "Pookie" Johnson

*"To love what you do and feel that it matters
—how could anything be more fun?"*

This quote by Katharine Graham, the late *Washington Post* publisher, is one of my favorites. This is how I feel about my passion for clowning in nursing homes and hospitals. I have no doubt that this is what I am meant to do at this time of my life. What a privilege! When I have heard others say, "You are so wonderful to do this," I feel a bit guilty as the blessings work both ways, and I receive double in return.

Or if someone says, "How can you do it? I couldn't stand the sadness," I don't think of it that way. I think of the personal attention and possibly fun and laughter I am bringing to a person in the nursing home that day. In some cases they may not remember me later, but for that moment I am making a difference in their life. I wish I could explain the high I feel after my visit with these people, several of whom have become my friends. Perhaps it is one of those things that are better "felt" than "telt"?

### *A Special Place in My Heart*

I clown for children and adults in hospitals and for the elderly in nursing homes. I love them all, but I do have a very special place in my heart for older people. The children I see are most often well taken care of and receive much 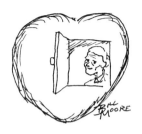 attention. It is the older folks who are often neglected or forgotten and need us so much. Also the staff and visiting families need encouragement and their hearts lightened.

I was a dog trainer and exhibitor since I was ten years old. As an adult I volunteered in nursing homes, visiting with my Golden Retrievers and a wonderful big old cat. Because of this, I had already become very comfortable visiting people in nursing homes before I became a clown.

I believe it is a great benefit if we are able to incorporate into our clowning the use of our natural talents that we already have, which is what I did with my dogs.

### *Finding My Niche*

When I first became a clown I spent a few years trying to find my "niche." I tried birthday parties, balloon sculpturing, stage performances, magic, and juggling. I think I thought I had to be able to do all these things in order to be a clown. For that reason, I really didn't become good at anything. I wanted to be a clown, but I just didn't know where.

Then I went to Clown Camp® and studied "Caring Clowning." I credit Richard Snowberg with all that I learned from him. He is truly the founding father of Caring Clowns.

I came to realize that nursing home and hospital clowning was where I belonged. It allowed me to use my personality and gift of caring for others. I prefer one-on-one interactions instead of performing on stage. I firmly believe that if I did not have this specialty I would not be clowning. There is a job for every clown, and this is mine. How fortunate I am to have found it.

# OUR STAFF
## INCLUDES

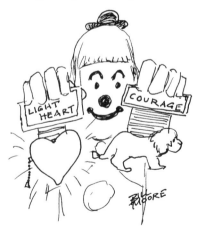

A CARING CLOWN

## My Dream

Now I realize that my heart and soul is in this mission. It is my dream that there will be a clown in every nursing home and hospital. It has become my privilege to teach classes in Caring Clowning in my home and at conventions around the U.S. and other countries. It is my mission to encourage others to become Caring Clowns.

## Take Heart!

It takes courage to be a Caring Clown. It takes courage to even drive down the street looking like that!

I clown by myself, as I do not have a caring clown partner. I think if you are going room to room, it is better to go as a single clown, one-on-one with a resident, giving them your undivided attention. Going as two clowns can become a performance between the two of you instead of just talking to the resident. Also, too many clowns can be overwhelming and confusing. But, when getting started, you could go with an experienced clown until you feel comfortable.

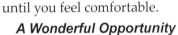

## A Wonderful Opportunity

Clowning in nursing homes is a wonderful opportunity to practice and gain confidence from experience performing in front of people. I know of no better way to become skilled at improvisation. You have to be prepared for anything that may happen.

It is pretty exciting to hear yourself come up with the most unexpected and funny thing that you have just said! I know that I became a better clown because of my experiences improvising as a Caring Clown.

### Getting Started

Choose a facility that is convenient for you. Contact the Activities Director and arrange for an appointment. Do not go in costume to that meeting. Explain what you would like to do. I think it is best to go on a regular basis, for example once a week or once a month.

This is your big chance to have your "name up in lights," listed on the monthly activity calendar! If you say you will be there, keep your word, unless you are ill or otherwise unable to go. Imagine the disappointment to the director and the residents if you did not show up when you said you would. You may be required to have a background check and an annual TB test.

### Fill Their Waiting Time

I know that it should be our rule to only go at a prearranged time, but there is one time that I personally break this rule. Because I have gone so many years to the same nursing homes and am known there, I have permission to drop in. If I have extra time in a clowning day, I sometimes stop at one of my nursing homes just before I know they are scheduled to serve lunch.

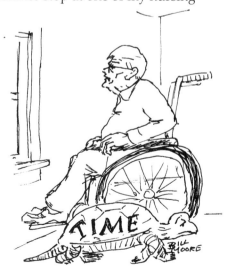

When the people are being brought into the dining room and waiting for their lunch to be finally served, it must seem like a very long wait for them.

This is a perfect time for me to drop in and do a little entertaining and visit. I leave as I see the food trays arriving.

### Have a Gentle Clown Face

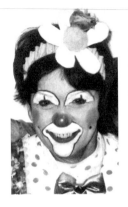

I like to use my full Auguste clown make up and costume when visiting nursing homes because I am most comfortable doing that, and sometimes it has started a conversation about the residents' memories of seeing clowns in circuses. It is very important to have a kind and gentle make up design.

I do not recommend visiting in a clown doctor costume because that can be too confusing to some residents.

Hospital clowns do not wear gloves because of infection control and being able to wash their hands. Although infection control is not as much of a concern in nursing homes, I do not wear gloves there either. There is a great value to touching. Sometimes I will hold their hand or gently rub their shoulder or back as I talk to them.

### Your Greatest Skill: Sensitivity

In Caring Clowning, sensitivity should be your greatest skill. As in all clowning we should "know our audience." You have to be able to assess what they are capable of understanding and enjoying. We must be sensitive to a person and situation and feel the moment. It is something that comes from within, being able to sense what to say or do. You develop that sense through experience. We all make mistakes, and that is our greatest teacher.

I am a Christian, but when I go to a nursing home I am very careful not to preach to the people that I see. However, if somebody mentions their faith, I will have a conversation with them about God.

### Going Room to Room

When I approach someone in a room, I always make eye contact first and say something like, "There's a clown here. Do you mind if I come in?" Many people can't see you from a distance or even realize what you are.

When I come up behind someone in a hallway I warn them by saying, "There is a clown behind you." I know that a clown is about the last thing they expect to see and I never want to scare them!

If there are visitors or staff members in the room, I have to be sensitive as to whether they need privacy or would welcome a diversion. Many times I have provided visitors as well as the resident a time of shared laughter.

When I enter a room, I like to look for something to comment on to start a conversation. If there are any decorations I say something about them. If there are photos on their bulletin board, it gives me an opportunity to talk about their families.

The main thing that I do on my visits is have a conversation with the residents. Many of them get few visitors and are lonely. A kind listening ear is one of the best things you can give them.

I don't ask people their name. Sometimes they don't remember and that would embarrass them. I look to see if their name is posted outside the door, and then I am able to call them by name.

### Performances

It is possible to go as a group and perform a short program in an activity room. Realize that perhaps only a few will understand what you are doing. You can't take it personally if you look out in the audience and many are asleep!

> In nursing home clowning, success is not measured in laughter and applause but by the hearts you have touched and the difference you have made at that moment.

Sometimes clowns think they have failed if they did not seem to get much of a response. However, if you got a smile, you may have gotten the best response that they can give you. You may have done something very good for them, but you will never really understand how you have affected them. You could have been extremely successful without realizing it.

In nursing home clowning success is not measured in laughter and applause but by the hearts that you have touched and the difference that you have made at that moment.

## Invite Children

If you are doing a show at a nursing home you may want to suggest that they invite children of the staff, grandchildren of residents, or students from a nearby preschool. The residents so enjoy seeing young children and hearing their laughter. It also gives you somebody to interact with, adding more fun.

## Be Careful with Balloons

Many nursing homes have a birthday party at the end of the month. This could be a time that one or a group of clowns would be welcome to come, of course by prior arrangement. I have made balloons at birthday parties, and the residents so much enjoyed watching me make them while I talked with each person. I make hats or animals to hold, but in both cases I am very careful not to inflate the balloons too full as they are more apt to pop. I don't want to startle or scare anyone.

## Theme Parties

The activity directors at nursing homes get event calendars that list things like National Ice Cream Day. They use them to get ideas for theme parties.

One time a nursing home asked me to visit on Emmett Kelly's birthday. My husband Bruce is a tramp clown so I volunteered him to do a show which was very successful because so many of them remembered seeing the original Emmett Kelly.

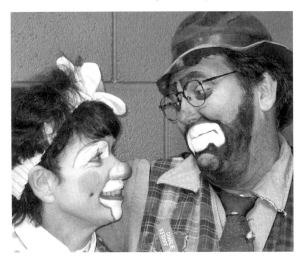

*Carole as "Pookie" with her husband Bruce "Charlie" Johnson*

### Circus Day

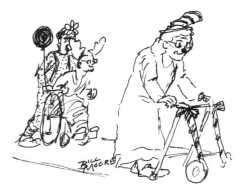

Another nursing home decided to have a circus day. The staff and some of the residents got dressed up. They decorated some tray tables like circus wagons and a few of the residents had decorated wheel chairs or walkers. I carried a tape recorder playing circus music and we had a circus parade up and down the halls.

Many nursing homes know about National Clown Week (August 1 to 7, see page 69) and are looking for clowns to visit during that time. This might give you a great opportunity to make your first visit.

### Your Greatest Prop: You!

Your patter*, your silliness, your personality is your greatest prop. Most important of all is the sharing of your heart. It is giving of ourselves with love.

I don't take many props to a nursing home, because few people can understand magic or puns and jokes. I always have a small magic trick in my pocket to use if a person would understand and enjoy it. For example, I use a tiny change bag with thumb tip blendo scarves. (*Shown at right—these can be ordered from clown suppliers.*)

### Puppet Fun

I rely mainly on a special puppet, which helps me to start an interaction, a contact, and make the resident feel important. I have a rabbit and a sheepdog puppet that are very lifelike. Sometimes a resident will believe that they are real, and I have to make the decision to either go along with them or say that it is a puppet. After all if we are having fun, what difference does it make? If they ask me if one is real, I sometimes say, "She thinks she is!"

*"Patter" is the words a clown speaks when using a prop or doing a routine.

## Stuffed Animals

Several friends give me new or nearly new stuffed animals, which I give to residents from time to time. I may carry one along with me as a prop, or a couple in a bag, and give it to someone I feel needs a little company. What is more wonderful than a soft teddy bear?

## Musical Instruments

I think a musical instrument would be a perfect prop to use in a nursing home. The residents love music, especially the old songs. If you can play only one song like "You Are My Sunshine" they will be impressed. They won't know that is all you can play.

As in everything we do, we must practice. I have been practicing the harmonica and ukulele. One of these days I am going to become a star. How many of us wish we had continued with the piano when we were a kid?

## If You Visit with a Dog

I don't always go as a clown when I visit nursing homes with my dogs, but you can certainly do both at the same time. My Golden Retrievers are big dogs, and I have felt it can be overwhelming for a resident to see a clown and a big dog at the same time. (Actually, I think the truth is that my dogs would get all the attention, and I would be jealous!)

Because I do this separately, I also feel that the residents get to see me twice and not even know it— once as a clown, and later as

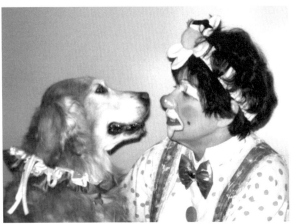

a human with a beautiful dog. A clown taking a smaller dog, dressed in a clown ruffle, doing some simple tricks could be a wonderful idea.

*"Pookie" with her dog Gracie.*

If you visit with a dog, it must be clean, trained, and have a record of current vaccinations. The dog should be a working partner with you, caring about people just as you do. My beloved Gracie is a perfect example of this. I have witnessed many times how she will sense and go on her own to the person who truly needs to see her. How precious she is to me.

If you are interested in doing pet visits you can get more information from the Delta Society at 875-124th Avenue N.E., Suite 101, Bellevue, WA 98005-2531. Their website is www.deltasociety.org. Email: info@deltasociety.org Their telephone number is 425-679-5500. Their *Team Training Course Manual* is currently $40.80 plus postage.

### My Wish for You

Clowning in nursing homes does matter. You make a difference one person at a time by bringing the gifts of listening and laughter to residents, lifting the spirits of visitors, and encouraging staff members. I love doing it.

I wish you the courage to make your first visit and hope that, after you experience how much fun it is, you will return again and again. Then you will bring my dream of a clown in every hospital and nursing home one step closer to becoming a reality. I would enjoy hearing from you.

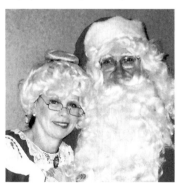

*To contact Carole see page 190.*

Also see Carole's encouragement to visit nursing homes as Santa and Mrs. Claus in Chapter 9 page 150.

*Carole and her husband Bruce as Mrs. Claus and Santa*

**National Clown Week** (cited on page 67) began in 1971 by U.S. Presidential degree which declared, "For surely the laugh-makers are blessed: They heal the heart of the world."

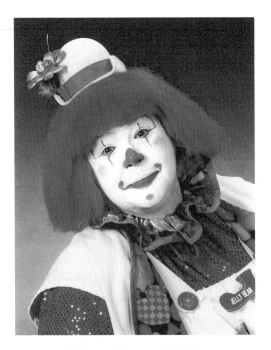

# Give Them TLC:
# Time, Listening and Caressing

By Janet "Jelly Bean" Tucker

How do I begin to tell you about my love for nursing home residents, or my philosophy in clowning for them, or about my thousands of special moments as I give Jelly Bean a chance to play with these elderly folks?

## *It's Play*

That's what it is—"play"—because scientists tell us we regress back to childhood ways the older we get. But the play goes beyond that to being the connection for laughter and memories for these elderly folks who are spending the rest of their days in a facility that can get pretty boring.

They have television, sometimes a game day with Bingo, sometimes a special event like a Valentine's party, but generally the days are long and very similar one after another.

### Here Comes
### the Clown!

And then, "Here comes the clown!" and one after another I meet residents who begin to tell me about their family, their recent trip to the doctor, and all the everyday stories they want to share with someone.

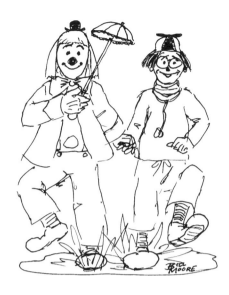

These stories soon turn into memories of the day they took their children to the circus or the day as a child they sneaked into the circus tent to see the show.

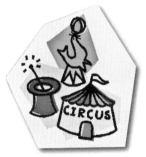

I hear about the fellow who once jumped aboard a train and rode like a hobo during the depression.

I know the ladies who remember Lou Jacobs and Emmett Kelly, a big favorite here in Indiana.

### Comparing Hospital Visits. . .

First I should give you my experience as far as the differences between a hospital clown visit and a nursing home clown visit. In a hospital, the patient is there for a relatively short time, generally is not feeling very well so needs a shorter visit from the clown, and has very limited space for any giveaways the clown might offer.

### . . . to Nursing Home Visits

In a nursing home, the residents are there for the rest of their lives, generally are feeling pretty good although somewhat bored, and have their own room or space to keep treasured mementos from the clown.

### Take Time Visiting

What do I do at a nursing home? Knowing that they are there to stay, I take my time visiting. I try to remember "TLC" which is Tender Loving Care, but I like to think of it as Time, Listening and Caressing when I visit the elderly.

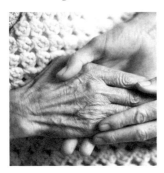

Take time to visit and to listen to them and always hold the little old hands gently or put an arm around a shoulder so they have some skin touch with the clown.

Again, this is very different from a hospital visit where the clown must be so aware of disease and infection control.

### Give Them "Love Lotion"

I have a bottle of hand lotion that I put a computer-generated label on saying "Love Lotion." I share the love lotion and put a bit on their hands and gently massage it in. I look into their eyes and talk with them as I'm applying the Love Lotion, and I take my time with each one in this special moment.

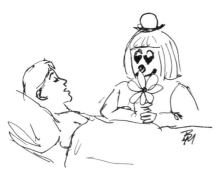

### Room Visits

I walk from room to room to see those who are in beds and sometimes do a little pocket magic trick or leave them a sticker or take an instant photo of them with the clown that they can keep.

### Activity Room Shows

I generally do a show in the activity room or dining room for those who can come out, either walking or in wheelchairs. The show has some puppetry, some audience-involvement magic where they get to wave the wand or hold the silks or say the magic words, and I do music. If it's a visit with my church group, we sing old hymns which I either play on the piano or use a CD. If it's a visit with my clown alley, I use some old songs with a banjo CD—things like "A Bicycle Built for Two" or "Harvest Moon" or "Has Anybody Seen My Gal."

For many years (until the facility was sold and merged with another home some distance away), I visited one particular nursing home every month and did a birthday party for all the residents who had a birthday in that month. I brought various gifts for each birthday person in that month, such as a box of tissues or footie socks or a Mylar helium balloon, or a bottle of hand lotion.

## Huggable, Comforting Gifts

The absolutely best gift I was ever able to give was the year I was blessed by a dear friend who was an executive with Dakin© Toys, and he gave me cases of stuffed animals to give to the residents. Those stuffed bears and turkeys and dogs and cats took up residence on their beds immediately, and many of the residents carried their animals around with them—soft, huggable, and very comforting.

In another home, I spent a year or so visiting those patients in the Alzheimer's unit. It started with a lady who hired me to do a birthday party for her mother who was in that unit. I had such a good time and such an alert response to what I did that the home asked me to continue my visits until, again, that unit was phased out and those people sent to another facility.

I learned that Alzheimer's patients still make connections with things they did often before the disease set in. The men spent hour after hour simply playing with remote controls. The ladies spent hour after hour folding little hand towels or playing with baby dolls. Ideal birthday gifts for the men had buttons to push and levers to move, while the ladies liked scarves and pretty hankies and fancy little dolls.

## Unusual Responses

It's important to realize that your clown may not get the response you do when you are with the general public or at a parade. One very strange story I can share will corroborate this truth. Some friends and I came in the door of a facility that was square in floor pattern with the nurses' station and dining room in the center and the rooms around the outside edge. As we began to visit in each room, one lady stayed right with us, screaming at us to leave and cursing at us loudly outside each doorway. She was very annoying, but some of the residents said she was always that way so we continued around the building.

Because of her noise and cursing and disruptive behavior, we decided we wouldn't do a show but would just do room visits and then leave. As we got to the door to exit, she went ahead, opened the door for us, and in a perfectly normal voice said, "Please come again soon. That was such fun!"

## Become a Special Memory for Them

Often during a show time, some of the people will nod off or have to leave the room for some reason. Don't take this personally as I've sometimes had those same people remember exactly what I did and request something to be repeated the following month. In every group, there is always someone who is alert and wants to participate so play to that person and become a special memory for them.

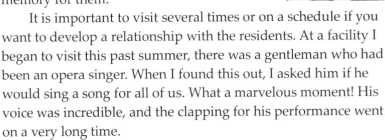

It is important to visit several times or on a schedule if you want to develop a relationship with the residents. At a facility I began to visit this past summer, there was a gentleman who had been an opera singer. When I found this out, I asked him if he would sing a song for all of us. What a marvelous moment! His voice was incredible, and the clapping for his performance went on a very long time.

The next time we came, he said he had been waiting for us and had thought of several songs he would like to sing for us. I suggested we do one "special" a month, and it has been a delight to hear him as well as see his enthusiasm for preparing for us. I'm certain he does not get many opportunities to share this talent, but it's become something we all anticipate now when we come.

## Ways to Involve Children

I'd like to share something I learned doing nursing home visits with my Sunday School children. As Department Head over the 1st through 5th graders, I schedule a nursing home visit about three to four times a year to a facility close to our church. While I generally don't go as a clown because I am in charge of the children, I use many of the same entertainment activities I use as a clown—songs, puppets, and magic tricks or skits.

On our first visit, the children were a bit apprehensive and held back from visiting with the residents. So on our second visit, I gave each child a paper with a list of things from A to Z and lines to be filled in with resident's names. A—person who once lived in Alabama; B—person who has a birthday this month; C—person who once owned a cat, D— person who once owned a dog . . . through to Z—person who once visited a zoo. The children now had a reason to ask the residents questions. They found out names. They found out facts about each person. They developed relationships. They wanted to return again soon because they had made some friends of these elderly people.

Since that time, I always open with an audience involvement activity for the children to personally meet the residents and become familiar with them before we start our show. It works equally well with our clown alley, and we always have a warm-up activity to meet and greet the residents when we arrive.

## More Blessings Than You Can Imagine

I've found that those days I set out to be a blessing to the residents in a nursing home are days I come home even more blessed. It's been said that, "You can't out-give the Lord," and that is truly proven when you begin to give your clowning to those in a nursing home or assisted living facility as the blessings come back to you in more ways than you can ever imagine.

*Visit Janet at* www.jellybean-clown.com/ *To contact her, see page 199.*

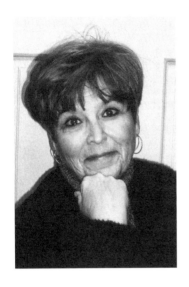
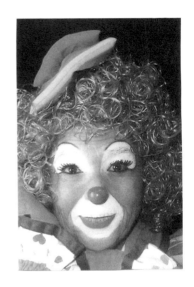

# Make It Fun

### By Judy "The Cute One" Barker

The first time I went out to clown was at a nursing home. I was overwhelmed by how receptive and how grateful they were that we had come to see them. Wow, what a wonderful way to start out clowning.

That was when I realized my passion for clowning. Today, when I teach hospital/caring clowning, I train them by going to nursing homes. Where else can you go that, no matter what you do, they love you unconditionally?

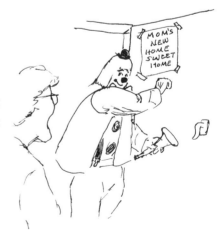

### *This Is Their Home*

Too many times we forget that this is their space and that we have been invited into their home.

There are not a lot of rules, but there are some common courtesies.

---

### Never Talk Down to Them

First thing to remember is never talk down to them. I remember one time I went to a birthday party for a little 99-year-old lady. Her great niece was in charge. She bends down to Auntie and says in a loud slow voice:

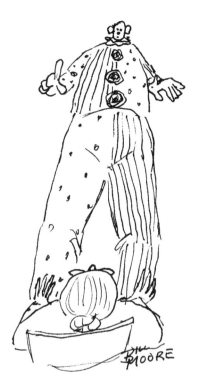

"THERE...IS...A... CLOWN...HERE...TO... SEE...YOU...TODAY. ARE...YOU...GOING... TO...LAUGH...AT... THE...CLOWN?"

The very alert 99-year-old lady turns to her great niece with an incredulous look and says, "If she says something funny I will."

I can't speak for the great niece, but Auntie and I had a great time that day and I certainly didn't make the mistake of talking down to her.

### Ask Permission and Accept "No"

If you are making a room visit be sure to ask permission to enter, and if they are non-responsive ask permission anyway. (You never know what they can hear.)

Be prepared that they may say, "No" and, if they do, then honor that decision. (There has been a time or two when I've not wanted someone in my home either.)

If you are invited in, then please be careful not to move, pick up or handle their personal items. But do look and observe the things around the room to use as a way of connecting with them.

### Begin a "Star-Studded" Conversation

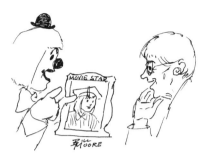

If I see pictures of family or friends, I'll ask if those are photos of movie stars.

Boy, is that the beginning of a conversation!

If you happen to be visiting with a person that is in a "different" world, sometimes it's nice to just go "there" instead of trying to drag them back into our world. If you listen, sometimes you can learn from someone else's history. Have fun and enjoy the moment with them.

### Make the Commitment to Connect

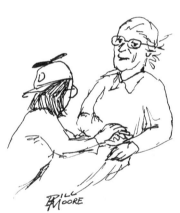

If you are going to give a show at a nursing home you need to make the commitment to connect. Too many people go and "do their show" and leave and have never really looked at the people nor touched them. I stress the importance of physically touching every single person when you get there and let them know that you are glad to be there and that you are going to entertain them and have fun.

### Make Skits More Visual Than Verbal

If you are going to do skits make sure that they are more visual than verbal because many residents have a hard time hearing. Make your movements exaggerated because even if they can't hear, they will still have fun watching.

Did you notice I keep using the word FUN???? That's your job as a clown ya' know. If you tell a joke or do a blow off * and they don't catch it, EXPLAIN it. (I happen to have several young friends for whom I have to explain jokes.)

*A blow-off is a funny or surprise ending to a skit.*

---

### Stir Up a Fun Skit

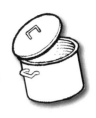

We do the skit called "Stew." The First Clown is stirring a big cooking pot. The Second Clown sees him stirring and says, "Can I stir?" "Okay," says the First Clown, "if you promise to keep stirring." The Second Clown stirs and then tastes and says, "Maybe this needs salt."

A Third Clown comes in and asks, "Can I stir?" Then he tastes and says, "Maybe it needs pepper."

Finally the First Clown comes back in, reaches into the pot, pulls out a pair of socks and says, "Thanks for doing my wash."

Usually the residents "get it" but occasionally they don't and if they don't I say, "Those silly clowns. The First Clown was washing his socks and the Second and Third Clowns thought it was stew" (and I pause to give them time to catch the joke) and then they'll laugh.

If the residents talk to you during the skit then use that in the skit—don't just ignore them. We did a skit about finding a dollar bill. In the very *next* skit I have to ask one of the clowns if he has any money. At that point a lady in the front hollers out, "I know he has a dollar 'cause I saw him when he found it on the floor." It changed our whole skit and it really kept us on our mental toes.

### Get Their Attention with Music

When we are setting up for a show, we'll play some of the songs of yesteryear and it always gets their attention. Sometimes they will come out of their rooms just to see what is going on in the recreation room or cafeteria or perhaps even the foyer.

Be prepared to do your show anywhere. Only one time did we have a stage. It was at a very expensive home with a beautiful theatre and seating for 50. Someone forgot to mention to the evening shift that we were coming, and we had five people in our audience. There were 10 clowns. Five clowns sat in the audience, one with each person, and five clowns performed. Then we switched. We got a standing ovation. Okay, at least 50 percent were "ovating."

## Do Things "with" Them

Make sure you involve your audience. It's important to do as many interactive things as possible. People are always doing stuff *to* and *at* but not *with* them.

I have musical instruments that we can use, but their favorite is a shaker made from a Doritos plastic hour-glass shaped container. Clean it and put some popcorn kernels in there and seal with a little glue. You can decorate anyway you like and "ta-dah!" you have a light, easy to hold musical instrument, and if someone gets really attached to it you can afford to give it to them.

### Easy Music Makers

I also get the great big jingle bells after Christmas when they are on sale and sew them onto elastic strips and put Velcro on them and they can easily be placed around their wrists and they don't have to hold it. They can just move their arms and make music.

### Create Theme Shows

Theme your shows with current events. (They watch a lot of TV.) Around Olympics time I had an Olympics theme. I made a torch out of foil, and I had them pass it off to each other.

Now, anyone who knows me is aware of how much fun I have with toilet paper. As soon as you pull out a roll, people know you are going to have a good time. So, I put down long strips of toilet paper for the "tracks" and had Olympic races. I also had a long strand of toilet paper for the "finishing line." I buy cheap medals that can be presented to the winners. I also give out long stem noses to the first, second, third, fourth, and fifth winners, etc.

*Place clown noses on the ends of artificial flower stems for "long stem noses" (at left).*

Around Easter I had an Easter hat parade. I gave them paper hats. (The pirate hats were their favorite.) We had a parade up and down the halls, and the people that were room bound could see us and enjoy.

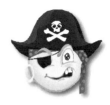

They always love chair dancing. For something different make it a prom theme. You could even use the same hats for the dress up. Ask them whose name they would like to put on their dance card. (I promise you someone will always say ELVIS—okay, maybe it's me—but they will shout out some great names.) Then we do our chair dancing. Remember, have FUN.

Late October I do a Halloween or Fall Festival show. You can make a lot of "costumes" by just having the "front" of some overalls or a funny dress and just "lay" it on the people or again put a little Velcro around the neck to hold it on.

Use hats, feather boas, scarves or anything the local Goodwill might have. Sometimes you can find cheap costumes after Halloween. They can even be kid's costumes since you are just laying them on and it doesn't have to fit. Make sure that everything is washable or something you can spray and disinfect.

Believe it or not even the men get into the costuming as long as you don't call it "dressing up." Anyone who doesn't want to do so can be a judge. You could even give out some little trophies or make up paper certificates—something they can show that they won. Of course you can have as many categories as you think up.

### Give Them Parts in Stories

Interactive stories are always good to get everyone involved. One of my all time favorites is The King With The Terrible Temper. (See this on pages 162-164.) I got this from the Saratoga Springs NY clowns and have been asked by the residents to do it again and again.

In fact one visit I did it three times. (Everyone wanted a part.) I use a tiara for the Beautiful Young Daughter, a crown for the King and a small crown for the Handsome Young Prince. I use a short stick horse that I bought for $3 for the Fiery Steed.

## "Jest" an Animal Story

I have a story that I wrote but unfortunately it is flying around in computer land which by the way is the REAL never never land. However, I can give you the "jest" of the story, and you can make up your own.

I buy the paper plates that are in the shape of faces of different farm animals. I think they also have plates with zoo animals and dinosaurs. Home Depot will give you the paint stirring sticks for free.

Glue or staple the faces onto the top of the sticks. They are easy for the people to hold, and everyone can see them.

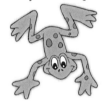

The story goes like this: Once upon a time there was an incredibly handsome frog. His name was Elmer. Now Elmer would go around his pad all day long going, "Ribbit, Ribbit, Ribbit." (Everyone says this together.)

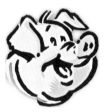

One day he went to see his friend the pig whose name was Hormel, and he would roam around his sty all day long going—at this point everyone will say, "Oink Oink" and you will say, "No, he said, 'Who, Who.'"

But what do you think the owl says? They say, "Oink Oink," and you say, "No, he said, 'It's dark up here.'"

Anyway, you make cardboard sayings for all the animals, and they all try to get their own words. The end of the story is that you go around and put the right words with the right animal. Sometimes the residents get confused, but then so do I and that's the fun part.

### Invite Them into Your Fantasy World

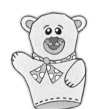

Puppets are great for visiting. Our elders are like children because they will come into your fantasy world if invited.

A lot of people take a dog or cat or monkey puppet. "Hi, what's your name?" they say to the resident. (Don't ask their name as they may be embarrassed because they can't remember.) YOU are a clown so make it FUN. (Hey, there's that word again.)

### Try a Different Approach to Puppets

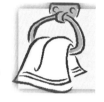

Try a different approach to puppets —something they don't normally see. It doesn't have to be elaborate. Get a washcloth and put eyes and mouth on it and introduce your "spineless" best friend who tends to be influenced by peer pressure since he has no backbone.

I also use this with kids when I talk about peer pressure and it's so ridiculous they all listen. I know what you are thinking, but if you are a beginner it's better to master the washcloth and then work up to the more professional bath towel.

### A Different "Therapy Dog"

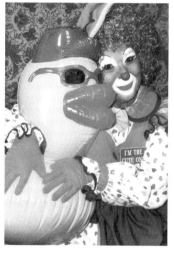

What can I say about Duke? Duke is a huge yellow blow up duck with sunglasses and a real attitude.

Here's the story. Duke is my Therapy Dog. Sometimes I ask the nursing home to advertise that a lady will be bringing her performing therapy dog. Then of course I walk in with this huge yellow duck.

I tell them I am very sorry but Duke will not be performing nor doing any therapy today. He was such a good therapy dog and then one day around Halloween he put on this duck costume and now he won't take it off. He used to do the most death defying tricks, but now when I take him with me he just sits there. So instead of DOING therapy, he now GOES to therapy.

I put him to the side, go on with the show and periodically I'll ask if anyone saw him move (because I'm hoping he'll perform). Occasionally, I'll have someone tell me that yes they thought he moved and once someone saw him do one of his tricks. Unfortunately, no one else saw it.

It had been a year since I had visited one particular nursing home, and when I got there they asked if Duke the Dog was with me.

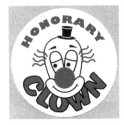

### Leave Them with Pictures

Because they have shared the joy of laughter with us, we make them honorary clowns. We give each one a red nose and take a photo of them with a clown.

Before you go to the home you want to make sure it is okay with the director to take photos. Always use a Polaroid because there are no negatives.

After explaining what we do with the film, the manager of our local store sells me the film at a discount rate. We also have people donate money for film in memory of a loved one. Almost all of the nursing homes have a Polaroid camera and film, so before you go ask them if they would like to take a photo of each resident with a clown. It's always nice if they'll use their own film.

### Give Them Something to Share

Pictures make your brain remember. The residents can relive your visit again and again. It seems like everything is brought to them, and people are always coming and telling them about the outside world, but the resident has nothing to share.

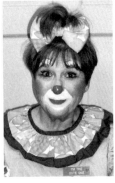

*As clowns, we are always changing to meet the needs of those we serve. For close-up visits, I am developing a modified clown face with no wig.*

Everyone has a need to give. You are empowering them by giving them a picture that they can share with others. They can say, "This is what I did today, and I can show you."

One home that we went to had the residents make frames out of popsicle sticks so they could put the photos in them. They had feathers and sequins and lots of tactile objects. The frames were beautiful, and the residents were so proud. Two years later and they still have them hanging in their rooms.

### Say Something Special to Each One

When the show is over, we go to each person and say, "Thank you for letting us come into your home." We try to say something special to *each* person before we leave, even if they are "asleep."

We've actually had people open their eyes and say thanks for coming when we had thought them non-responsive. Remember: Never make assumptions and always work hard to get as much response as you can from a person, even if it's just to see a toe tapping to music or a small smile at the absurdity of your famous talking washcloth.

### Don't Forget the Staff

Remember to clown with the staff. They have hard jobs. It is important for you to share relief through humor. One person can make a difference.

The whole nursing home reflects the attitudes from the top on down. I can always tell how excited the residents are going to be by how excited the recreational director is about our visit. I also do continuing educational programs for Nursing Home and Assisted Living Directors. I want them to see the difference a good attitude can make in their staff as well as their residents.

### The Difference You Make

I've been told and I have seen the difference that clowns make by bringing laughter into the nursing home. It's a place where you can give a lot and yet receive back twice as much. The distinctiveness of nursing home clowning is that, no matter what you do, they love you. With this recognition comes an awesome responsibility. It's a responsibility to be the best clowns we can be

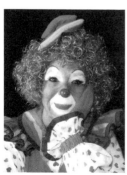

and do the best shows we can produce. They are our beloved elders. They say you can tell a lot about a society by the way they treat their young and old. Our performance, our compassion, and our commitment to excellence will show who we are—as clowns and as human beings.

*Judy Barker is founder and president of A Healthy Humor Clown Unit, Inc. that teaches therapeutic clowning. To contact her, see page 187.*

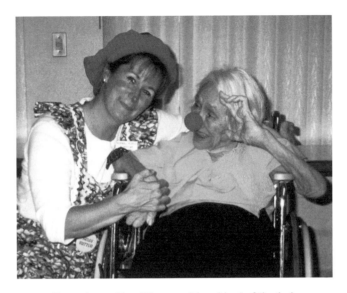

*Pancakes with a 98-year old resident of the Luis Elizondo Nursing Home in Monterrey, Mexico.*

## Treasure Their Uniqueness

### By Susan "Pancakes" Kleinwachter

"Someday, we're all going to get old."

I remember hearing that many times from my elders and guess what? They were right! What I didn't seem to think about or realize when I was younger is the amount of treasures and stories each individual person holds and can share with the world. Every person has a story to tell and possesses a uniqueness about them that makes them special.

That's why I love entertaining in nursing homes so much, because I am fortunate to have met so many wonderful people there that have become close in heart and have shared so many stories with me.

I prefer to entertain in a community room setting. To me, this gives the residents a place to be and creates an atmosphere for setting the stage before I start my shows.

Here are a few suggestions I can share with you in order to make your entertaining there have a deeper connection.

### Think of Themes

Before I book a show, I offer several ideas for different themes. Sometimes a holiday theme is good and other times I make up theme shows in order to offer something they have never seen before that would be interesting, fun and memorable. Creativity and activity are the key ingredients for this. I try to have a nice mixture of music, magic, audience participation, games, and songs. I also have a wonderful theme book that I get a lot of ideas from.

### Send Them Your Picture

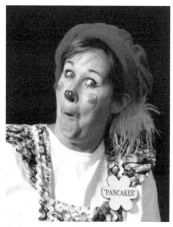

After I book the show through the activity director, I forward a flyer with my picture on it so it is a constant reminder to the residents that I am coming to visit. This technique builds an excitement and gives them something to look forward to.(Think of how it would be if you seldom got to leave your house and had few visitors or had scheduled visits on the weekends only from your family members.) Now it is easier than ever to create your own flyers from your computer and print on decorative paper.

### You're on a Roll

When I arrive, I check in with my contact and begin unloading my car. It is a wise idea to have a wagon or some type of device with wheels to help you walk with your equipment, as the main community room can be far from the entrance. Also, handicap parking and wheel chair accessibility take up much of the front entrance spaces.

Many times it takes the residents a while to get to the community room or for enough assistants to help them get there. This is why announcing your arrival early is good. It allows plenty of time for both you and the attendees to come together.

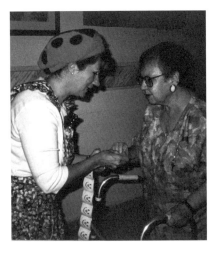

*Pancakes distributes stickers at the DuPage Convalescent Center in Wheaton, Illinois.*

*She never places stickers on wheel chair arms, walker handles, medical apparatus, bulletin boards or any equipment. She often places them on index cards and autographs them.*

If you are on a tight time schedule, you could ask that everyone be in the room by a particular time before you get there. My favorite time to entertain is right before lunch when energy levels are at their best.

### "Meet and Greet" Creates a Bond

I always like to take five minutes to meet and greet the residents in person and shake their hands or pat their shoulders gently. I want to make sure they know how glad I am to meet them and have them at the show. I want to validate their interest which creates an instant bond for conversation afterwards.

A key point to consider is the length of time they are able to sit still. Remember that many of them nap or take medications that make them sleepy. Many just plain need to be involved.

### Speak Slowly and Use Large Props

Your distance from the audience needs to be close-up because many of them can't see well or hear well. Your props need to be large and high in the air for them to see. Speaking a little slower will give them a better opportunity to process what you have said or respond to what you asked them to do.

I remember back in my earlier days of nursing home entertainment, when seeing them sleeping during the show made me feel I was doing uninteresting bits. In fact, one of the residents they wheeled in was sleeping when they brought her in, slept through the whole show and woke up after it was all over. She came up to me personally to thank me for the best show she ever was at!

I have never woken up a sleeping resident!

Since I am not familiar with what is going on in their lives, it's best to let them get their rest and sometimes it just happens to fall upon them during your show.

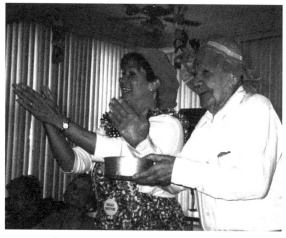
*Pancakes leads music with a resident.*

It's also a great idea to have the nursing home assistants there so they too can enjoy the show and get a break from the stress of life. After all, it's our job to entertain everyone.

### Fun and Easy "Tap Dancing"

One of my favorite shows to do is a "tap dancing" number with the residents and staff (while the residents are sitting in their chairs). I take canning jar lids around which I have glued elastic bands in order for their feet to fit inside. The lid portion is underneath their shoe.

We all do a "chorus line" number together. The noise created from the metal lid against the metal wheel chair foot is awesome! If they are not in a wheel chair, I use a tipped chair on an angle for their platform.

This set up time takes a few minutes; however, I make jokes and conversation with them as I go around the room and get everyone situated. For example I say, "I am checking to see if you are Cinderella and this lid fits!" or "I'm thinking your foot size and my clown shoe size are the same—size 22, right?"

This show brings the most smiles. The response from the music and tapping creates fun and giggles from the little effort they have to put into it.

After the show is over, I thank everyone individually once again for their participation and efforts. I also invite them to stay longer if they wish for what I call "KleinTime." (This is actually a time where we can all get to know each other better or share stories of their past.)

## A Cuddly Rabbit Draws Them Out

If I use my live rabbit, "Mr. Marshmellow," in the show, this would be the time they could pet him, ask questions about him, hold him and share some cuddles. He is 12 years old and extremely gentle and calm. Since he is so soft and cuddly, most all the residents enjoy their private one-on-one time with him.

I have seen many residents that were mentally in another world while I was visiting. When I brought my rabbit around for them to pet him, they became a whole new person, alive with expressions and smiles. It is amazing to see this transformation!

The hardest part of leaving the residents after the show is the question they often ask "When will you be coming back?"

I hope to some day start a resident's storytelling program where we could have video interviews about their past experiences that are recorded from the residents and use it for a reading program in the grade schools. Maybe even create a residents' adoption so the residents always have someone they could write to and communicate with outside the nursing home.

*Susan's website* www.KleinTime.com *offers supplies for nursing home clowns. To contact her, see page 192.*

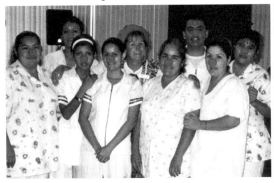
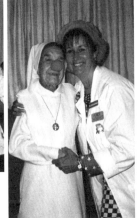

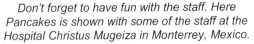
*Don't forget to have fun with the staff. Here Pancakes is shown with some of the staff at the Hospital Christus Mugeiza in Monterrey, Mexico.*

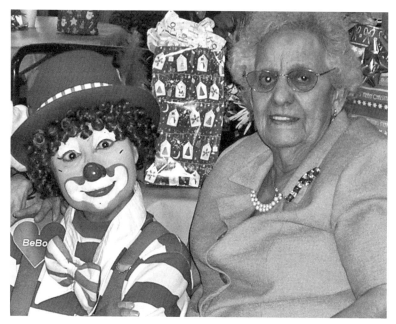

*Aurora "BeBop" Krause is shown with her mother, Angelita P. Gonzales, 84, at the Mount Carmel Assisted Living in Corpus Christi, Texas, where "BeBop" performed for the Christmas Celebration.*

# How Could I Not Be Here?

By Aurora "BeBop" Krause

It's true that nursing homes are not the places that many people enjoy visiting. Many times we hear that the sights and smells are hard to handle.

### Focus on Their Eyes

It is also true, however, that if we stay focused on the eyes of those residents we pass in the hallways and the patients we visit and perform for, these smells and sights become nonexistent.

I don't know for sure if the eyes are the windows of our souls. I do know that it is the look in their eyes that can make us forget the outside world. If we acknowledge their need for touch, attention and compassion, these residents will respond with a

> **It is the look
> in their eyes
> that can make us forget
> the outside world.**

grateful and receiving heart. As a performer and a caring clown, I could not ask for a greater reward.

I have been clowning at assisted living and nursing homes for the past eleven years. Many times I'm tired and not really interested in getting "into clown" but I do, and the minute that "BeBop" walks into the first patient's room or begins a performance, I think to myself, "How could I have thought not to be here?"

Their eyes light-up, the smile comes across their face and they know I'm there just for them. My approach is always the same, one of gratitude and generosity. I'm grateful to be here, and I hope I can make things better.

### Wake Up Their Memories

Nursing home residents have memories that make them smile and put joy in their hearts, but they need someone or something to wake-up the memories and bring that smile to their faces. These moments serve as a pleasant distraction that breaks through the illness and the loneliness…Sooo, in walks the clown.

It is the caring clown character that we have developed with love and compassion that first greets the residents—a caring clown that creates a warm curiosity that interests their heart and opens the door for a joyful encounter.

### Caring Comes First

One very important thing we must remember when clowning in an assisted living or nursing home environment is that we are there for the residents not for ourselves.

From the time we enter we focus on each individual and set aside our prepared performance, magic tricks and routines. First let them know how much you care and how glad you are to see them. There will be time to do your performance and share some fun later. First provide them with the time they need to take you in and absorb the attention that you're sharing.

### When to Schedule

Most of the time, when clowning at an assisted living or nursing home I work directly with the activities director. They will request a one-hour performance, room-to-room visits or both. For a one-hour performance I'm usually scheduled from 10:30 to 11:30. The residents will have been gathered in the dining room by 10:30 and therefore are ready for lunch at 11:30 when my show is over. This works well for the staff, and I can work with this time-frame.

I may also do a performance in the afternoon from 3:30 to 4:30, which serves the same benefit for their evening dinner time.

When you visit an assisted living or nursing home on a regular basis, the residents become familiar with what to expect and look forward to some music and fun. Because they like routine, I always begin and end the shows the same way.

### What I Do in Performance Shows

I begin with some upbeat music that they're familiar with and I end with some well known gospel songs that they know the words to and can sing along. In between, I include a combination of music and dancing with some comedy magic and comedy routines. As long as a resident is willing and able to participate I let them join in.

Wheelchairs are never an obstacle; I hold their hands and dance away. Many times I exaggerate my dancing and ask them to please slow down for me; this makes them laugh and we all enjoy the fun.

Examples of some excellent props to incorporate with music, which also encourage participation, are inflatables such as beach balls, musical instruments, baseball bats and balls. These are also easy to wash and keep clean between shows.

In closing the show, and with the permission of the activities director, I always end with a couple of good old gospel songs that they know the words to such as "He's Got the Whole World In His Hands."

### Special Considerations

It's true that many residents have poor eyesight and hearing. For this reason any assisted living and nursing home entertainment should be put together with some special considerations. If your show has music, insure that it is away from your audience, preferably behind you. Feedback from the

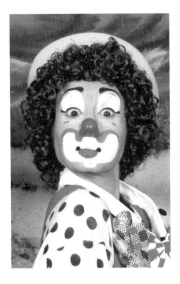

speakers can be very uncomfortable to those residents wearing hearing aids.

### Make Clear Expressions

Whether you are entertaining room to room or in the form of a performance:

> * Prepare your routines to be performed slowly.
> * Use large props.
> * Make clear movements and expressions.

### Personalize Each Interaction

I make it a point to get close with every resident in attendance and share some words either before, during or after each show.

I squat down to their level and hold their hands gently and tell them I'm glad to see them and hope that they're having a good day.

Attendance for your performance will vary from 20 to 80 residents for a variety of reasons. Room-to-room visits are done if they're requested. Many times residents who have been regulars at my previous shows are no longer able to leave their rooms so I'll make visits to their rooms because they'll know I'm there and I know they would enjoy a visit from BeBop. I always find them to be grateful for the visit.

### Adapt to Different Audiences

There are several things I have learned from clowning for an older audience. There is a difference in the audience at a nursing home and those in an assisted living environment. The nursing home audience is more passive and sedate while the assisted living audience is more active and more likely to participate.

Focus on what would be entertaining to them as an older audience in regards to the music and routines you'll perform. Impressing them with exceptional slight of hand or using the latest gimmick is not necessary—you are there because you care.

---

## Include Family and Staff

I make a special effort to include family members or the staff in my shows whenever possible. The residents enjoy this and it allows for some lighthearted and fun interaction away from the daily medicines and routines. Give a loving thought to every situation and share joy with an open heart and your visit or performance will be a success.

It is difficult not to notice the sad and lonely faces you will see at an assisted living or nursing home. Emotionally you will be affected by the love and attention missing in these elderly people's lives.

When this situation gets me down, I remember a great quote from Thomas Jefferson who said, "He does most in God's great world who does his best in his own little world."

We may never know if we make a small difference in someone's life if even for a moment but these are some of the comments I have heard from some of the nursing homes I've visited:

"Thank-you for being here today. It was good to see a smile on my mother's face again."

"Tell whoever sent you that I said thank-you. I enjoyed it very much."

"Don't ever stop coming here. You make us happy."

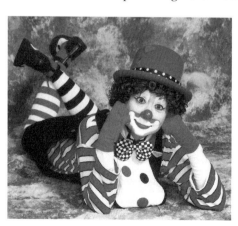

I will continue to clown at assisted living and nursing homes as long as my big clown shoes continue to take me there.

It is a privilege and a blessing to see the bright smiles on the faces of the elderly when "BeBop" simply walks into their world.

To contact Aurora, see page 193.

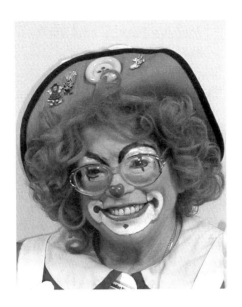

## Making Them Feel Special

By Carol "Blossom" Kay

Nursing home visits are amazing because we find folks in many different places in their health walk. The fit and able usually know when Blossom is arriving and they meet her right at the door and vie for the status of carrying any gear they can get their hands on.

It isn't necessary, but that's the very first place a clown can assist someone in feeling "special." Feeling special, loved, cared for and entertained is what Caring Clowning is able to accomplish.

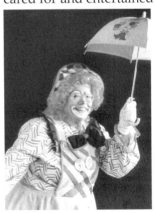

Blossom first goes to the "gatekeeper"—be it a nurse, receptionist or secretary—to announce her arrival. Once that's done, a little fun with them is the first order of business.

### Walk-Arounds

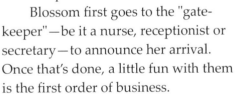

Blossom usually has a walk around in her pocket, a fancy balloon to give away, a puzzle or a sticker. This year the staff have been looking mostly for the sticker "IYQYQR." The runner-up is the nametag with "I SUFFER FROM HUMOROIDS."

A popular one with the residents is the sticker that looks like a band aid with a happy face in the ccntre. These sometimes go on clothing but mostly on walkers, canes and bedside tables. Reading my buttons and figuring out what they mean is like a competition in the common rooms.

### Mouth Coil Fun

There, too, when a group is gathered, I'll often grab a Kleenex tissue and start coughing a lot until I'm well noticed. Then I do a very long white mouth coil, first wrapping it around me, then a wheelchair, then one of the staff and we get all tangled up. The residents love it.

### Heart-Y Exercise

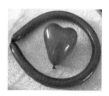 Then I'll hand someone in a chair a 260 balloon tied into a circle and ask someone to hold it out for me and then start tossing a heart through it and see if they can catch it. This gives the residents some exercise and good laughs.

### Change Bag Surprises

Blossom also likes doing tricks with the change bag like the three ropes becoming Tide 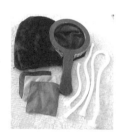 and the wee silk scarves becoming a  large silk with them all joined together at the end of the magic.

These are good to do because the residents don't have to touch anything —just say the magic words—so we have no concerns about passing germs with the clowning gear. Blossom looks for things that she can handle and then just show it at punch line time.

One hilarious activity is to approach someone and enquire if they've been asked to provide stool samples sometimes and they almost all have. Then I tell them that my dentist even asks for them now and that I never know when someone's going to ask me for one and it's a real bother. However, not to worry, I carry mine around all the time in my clown pocket. Wanna see it? Doctors often tell me, "NO." Nurses and residents are more curious, but guests like it even more.

Playing with the guests, adults and children alike, is really a favourite because I feel that if they have fun visiting the elderly and grandparents each time, they may come back more often. I reach into my pocket and pull out a wee black film container with STOOL SAMPLE printed on it, very official like. Inside is you know …a tiny doll house sized wooden stool! It sure does make folks laugh. That raises their endorphin levels.

### Mirroring Their Picture

Then I go up to complete strangers and ask their name and say, "My goodness, I have a picture of you in my pocket." They say, "Oh no you don't." They think just because I've never met them that I couldn't be carrying around their photo. Then I pull out a piece of wood about the size of a playing card with the words "MY NEWEST FRIEND'S PICTURE" then turn and show it to them saying, "Now tell me, isn't that a perfect likeness of you in the picture?" and sure enough it is. It's a mirror of course.

I also do the mirror on a piece of wood with one side having writing that says it's the clown's ID (or the senior's.) Then I look puzzled for a minute and turn it over only to see a wee mirror. I look in and say, "Well that's so true, IT IS ME!"

### Walking Around the Block

I also have in my pocket another piece of wood. I take it out of my pocket and ask someone to help me. Someone that is walking (even in a walker) will do. I ask them to take my arm and walk with me three times around the hunk of wood. I ask them to please count to three so we know when we're finished.

Then I thank them very profusely for helping me with my doctor's orders for the week. I tell them that the doctor said I was to find a friend and go for a walk around the block three times  each day! Before they can hit me with the block, I hand out FREE B's, GRAY V's, HICK E's and the like.

Occasionally I'll mention that I haven't had time for lunch and pull out a plastic banana and proceed to unzip it and pull out a real peeled banana and eat it!!!!! Not in front of children ever—that's a no-no.

### More Ideas

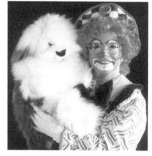

I also do rope tricks, squeaker tricks, chicken tricks, disappear things into thumb tip tricks, do balloon storytelling, balloon sculpturing and face painting. Staff are usually game to start off the face painting modeling, but soon the ladies want to all be butterflies or princesses, just like their younger counterparts. Men want to be pirates. I wonder why?

Visiting days where families are invited are one of the best days for balloons and face painting as the seniors love to see their grandchildren having fun. Whatever you do with the grandchildren is really good for the older folk to watch and participate. They don't hear children laughing near often enough.

Changing into bumblebee costumes and carrying a singing bumblebee cheers them up as well. Wearing a Santa Hat and carrying a singing moose; being all in red for Valentine's Day with cuddly teddy bears—all make their days different and special. When you go with any regularity, being seen in different costumes allows them to know that you're dressing up special JUST FOR THEM.

Just a wee hint! If you're face painting and forget your brushes, the personal care foam toothbrushes work quite well in a pinch.

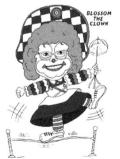

Hugs and Blessings to you all as you take some new ideas for visiting ME when my day comes to be in that chair or walker.

Blossom The Clown "The Blooming Idiot"
www.blossomtheclownbandb.com
Bradford, Ontario, Canada.

*To contact Carol, see page 191.*

# Treat Them As "Family"

By Curt and
Diana Patty
a.k.a. "Handy Andy"
and "Blossom"

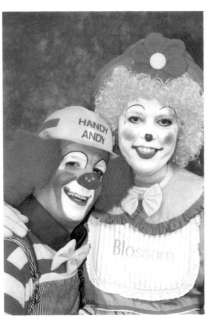

Nursing homes, veteran's homes and rehabilitation facilities are wonderful places to visit and share God's Love using the tools of clowning, puppetry and illusions.

In places like this, you may be an individual's only visitor in a very long time. A few things to remember:

### Treat Them as Your Own Relatives

These wonderful individuals may be here for different reasons (medical, physical, or mental afflictions) but they are someone's mother, father, grandparent, or child. Treat them as your own relative.

### Choose Music from Their Era

Be prepared. Know what era of individuals you will be meeting with. For example, come with a common song of the 1940's and 1950's era, not today's music. Bring a few different types: jazz, country, rock or swing and know the music to sing or dance a little with them.

They will hear it, and it will take them back to when they were young and dating or just married. Or it may take them back to times as a child—happy wonderful times in their life.

### Teach Balloon Twisting

Working with a group, teach them to twist balloons. This will help them with their dexterity—working their hands similar to what a physical or occupational therapist would do in their sessions. But check with the supervisor first for approval for latex precautions and for doctor approval that this will not interfere with any other treatments they may be receiving.

### Give Stuffed Animals

Collect small stuffed animals. New would be great, but if they are used and in good condition get them cleaned. This could be their only friend to keep them company. Help them to give it a name and keep it fed. This sounds childish, but there are times this will be appropriate.

Another thing to do is get a Polaroid type camera to take a picture of you and the resident. Leave the picture with them. Some individuals will treasure this photograph as you may be their only visitor in a while. Get permission from the person in charge before doing this.

### Important "No No's"

DO NOT promise anything to any patient, as you may not know if you can deliver.

There are three NO NO's <u>not</u> to talk about: sex, politics and religion. (If you are going there to do a religious service, then it is appropriate because the residents will know in advance what you are doing and can choose whether to participate.)

### Touch Gently and Avoid Spreading Germs

The nursing home is in many ways similar to the hospital setting with the exception that often the nursing home person needs a gentle touch.

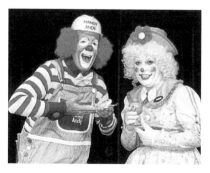

Care should be taken with the props you use to avoid spreading germs from one person to another.

Remember, you can change the world, one person at a time.

*Curt and Diana Patty's Clown Gadget Store offers easy to clean caring clown props appropriate for nursing homes. Visit their website at* www.clowngadgetstore.com *To contact them, see page 196.*

# Equip Them with Gags, Gifts and Giggles

By Tammy "Hugz" Miller

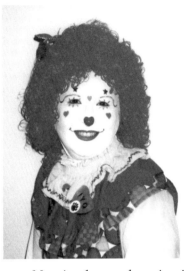

Maybe you are reading this information as a refresher or reference book and have been clowning in this setting for a long time. Maybe you are reading this as a newer clown and are trying to decide what you can do in the nursing home setting. The list of possibilities is endless and only limited by your imagination.

Nursing home clowning is often much closer, more one on one, and the activities can be on a smaller scale. Group skits and activities are also fantastic in the nursing home, but you do not always have the luxury of having everyone in the same room, so being equipped for the one on one can offer the greatest reward.

### Creative Give-Aways

Perhaps you are trying to decide WHAT you can do. In our clown group we have some of the most creative (that may be a politically correct way to say CRAZY!) people when it comes to little give-a-ways you can play with then leave with the residents.

Some are really corny—literally! For example, a small match box with a cover that reads, "Chicken Dinner" and inside you find 3 kernels of corn—now that's CORNY! Or a small plastic bag with a few pieces of straw and a note that reads, "Do it Yourself Straw Hat." Or one of my favorites—a small metal washer and a piece of cloth with a note that reads, "Washer and Dryer." These are examples of inexpensive gags that you can use, laugh at with the residents, and then leave for them to share the joke with others.

Other props that can play well in a nursing home include small musical instruments. I have a small plastic violin that can play either automatically or as I touch the strings. This can be good for pretending that you can play a song but do poorly, then push a button and let the instrument play by itself.

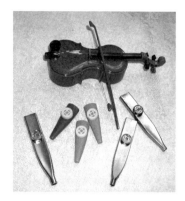

Violin or kazoo playing is fun because it gives the resident an opportunity to interact with you the clown. Plastic kazoos can be bought at a very low cost for you to leave.

Experience has taught us that music, especially the songs from the 40's and 50's, is extremely popular with nursing home residents to sing in both small and large groups. You can find some popular songs and lyrics in your library, talking with family and friends and on-line. You don't have to have a large repertoire; just learn two or three songs, even if it is just one or two verses that everyone can sing along.

Another inexpensive item is a "photo album" of colorful cartoons—the more colorful the better. Leave off the captions and create your own with the residents.

Rubber chickens, feather dusters, colorful balloon sculptures (get permission for balloons from the facility first)—all these can help you connect in the nursing home. The cognitive level of your participants will help guide you in the right direction for some of the gags and props you can use.

### Design Your Own Puzzles

Puzzles are another item in your bag of tricks, from a simple crossword puzzle or word search, to the more complicated puzzles, such as Sudoku. As a clown you can have fun starting the puzzle and let the resident finish it after you leave.

You can easily design your own puzzles at many web sites offered for free, or you can ask someone else to help you. These sites allow you to put in your own words and the puzzle is automatically generated. If you do a search for "make your own puzzle," you will have quite a few from which to choose.

You should consider leaving the answers just in case—you don't want to RAISE the stress level from your visit.

*See Tammy's insight on humor on pp. 14-17. To contact her, see page 195.*

# Listen with Love

## By Cathie "Periwinkle" Degen

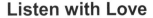

I approach Nursing Home Clowning similarly to what I do in the hospital. I do a lot of listening. I always try to hold their hands or maybe lightly squeeze their arm when I am talking with the residents.

Sometimes I bring a book of short stories like a *Reader's Digest* and get a small group of residents around a round table so I can interact and read to them. I try to find something that they can relate to.

One time I read a story about buttons and several women talked all about when they used to make clothing and used all types of buttons.

Sometimes, with permission, we will have snacks. I find that sometimes all some of the residents need is someone to talk with them or ask questions about their lives. I keep my clown make-up very low key.

I have also clowned in the Alzheimer's units. I usually bring music with me—something from their generation or something soft. I will dance with the residents or wheel them slowly around in the chairs. And those who can not walk or wheel, I will go to them and just take their hands and sway with them to the music.

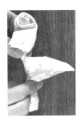

I also make napkin roses and give them out to those I know won't eat them. (For directions on how to make the napkin rose at left, turn to page 184.)

*To contact Cathie, see page 189.*

## Keeping Their Sunny Side Up

### Trudy "Birdie" Stryker

Everyone has probably heard of the cat puppet and cat scans but "Birdie" carries fill-able Easter eggs and does "egg-ams." I pass the egg over and around the resident and then crack it open, for a prize inside—a sticker or feathers, etc.

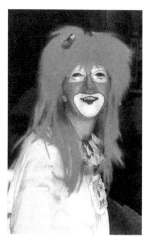

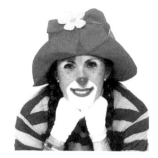

One of our clowns, Tera "Marty Pants" Bush (at right) carries a handheld doorbell and rings it for permission to enter people's rooms. It's fun because it gives residents a doorbell to hear and complete control on whether we visit with them.

*Trudy "Birdie" Stryker*

We've also found that anything musical is a big hit.

Another of our clowns, Kathleen "Posie" Leon, leads a group time with letting each resident pick from clown hats, wigs, etc. Then a group photo is taken. They love that. Care must be taken then to wash everything shared.

*To contact Trudy, see page 199.*

## You Never Know How You May Affect People

### By Brian "DR. Briny" Black

I do what I call my "mini-magic matinee" with the residents, staying about five minutes with each one and then moving on to the next. One time I met a woman who was extremely rude and obnoxious and I wanted to leave after one minute but I decided to stay and listen. I wound up staying two and a half hours and she turned out to be the nicest lady you'd ever want to meet.

I've learned that you don't always know how you may affect people. One time a nursing home director asked me for my clown picture because he said one of the residents had requested that it be placed on his casket at his memorial service. I was shocked. So you just never know.

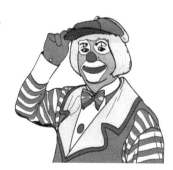

*To contact Brian, see page 188.*

# Elevating the "Humour Quotient" in Your Care Facility

## A Fun Resource
### By Karen "Rootin' Tootin' Newton" Baxter

*Karen has many pages of excellent ideas.*
*To learn more, contact her at the address on page 188*
*or see her ideas on this book's website at:*
www.angelfire.com/planet/nursinghomeclowning/

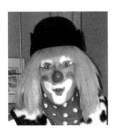

Recently, our Volunteer Director at our local Care Facility for Elders, indicated only a nucleus of residents turned out for activities. If your care facility suffers from the same malady, perhaps it's time to turn up the "HUMOUR" quotient in your building. If activities are meaningful, purposeful, and FUN, residents will come! If not, meet them where they're at. There is no evidence of any elder, in the last moments of life, wishing they'd had less FUN and LAUGHTER in their life! Some suggestions:

**Weekly Visit from the "Red Nose" Transplant Team**. Select several lucid residents and volunteers who would like to be part of the Team. No experience required, just a sunny disposition! They could sport colorful bibs, or bow ties, or hats, or jackets, and a "red" nose for easy identification. Their mission: to visit as many residents and staff as possible during their visit and spread chuckles and cheer!

An inaugural activity might be to plant a **RED NOSE TRANS-PLANT** in a high traffic area. Pot a branch from a dead tree and place a RED NOSE at the end of each branch. Place a sign at the base of the tree, for example: Studies have shown it to be true, when you "pick your nose," you can't be blue! So "pick your nose" and we guarantee, your heart will fill with giggles and glee!

Have the team put together a **"WACKY WIT" Wagon**, stocked with stickers, rubber chickens, cartoons, jokes, Wacky Words of Wisdom, silly props, Red Skelton and I Love Lucy videos, "Feel Good" movies. Example: The "morning paper." (Toilet paper on a paint roller).

**Post a Madcap Menu of the Day,** example: Eggs Funny Side Up, Light Snacks (light bulb in baggie), Light Lunch (light bulb in a lunch bag).

**Joke Jars**. Invite all who enter the facility to enter your weekly Joke Contest and submit it to the Joke Jar. When a humour break is needed, pull out a joke. At the end of the week, choose the "Joke of the Week" and post it on the "Joke of the Week" board. Weekly prizes consisting of free "B's" can be handed out! Or invite residents to design funny, silly fridge magnets to be distributed as prizes. *For more on Karen, see pages 138, 160 and 188.*

---

# Chapter 7
# Clowns in Ministry

One need not be "religious" or of any particular faith to clown with love and care in a nursing home. So why have a chapter on "clowns in ministry?" For one primary reason:

### To Connect with Many Residents

This book emphasizes connecting with your audience and being sensitive to where they are. For many in the nursing home generation, Christian faith is the bedrock of their lives and they speak openly of God. When you ask them what they'd like to sing, they often request hymns. Many residents remember the words to the Lord's Prayer or the 23rd Psalm even when other memories fade.

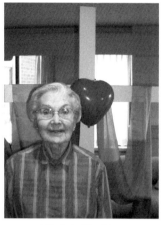

*Virginia Rackley,
a resident at The
Fairways at Brookline.*

The nursing home clown must never "mug" the vulnerable resident with their own religious views or interpretations. One is a clown, not a preacher and many residents are of different faiths. One tries to "speak" the love of God through one's actions.

But in addition, there can be times when your clowning can incorporate lighthearted messages *about* the love of God. The staff may even ask you to provide such programs in the community room or in weekly worship services offered in most facilities.

If you serve in this special outreach or wonder what it might be like, this chapter offers you some ideas. If you clown *because* of your Christian faith, this chapter may connect you with some others who feel called by God to clown.

In his book *Wishful Thinking: A Seeker's ABC* (Harper, San Francisco, 1993) Frederick Buechner writes, "The place God calls you to is the place where your deep gladness and the world's deep hunger meet."

For many clowns in ministry, that place is a nursing home.

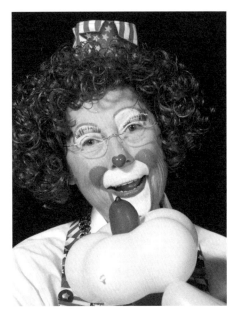

# Besides God, Know Whom You Are Serving

By Donna "Spangles" Shuster

There are various types of Homes that may call on you to entertain their residents. From Independent Living, to Assisted Living, to Skilled Nursing Homes, you must have a clear vision of your perspective audience. Knowing the TYPE of home and the general environment will greatly determine the program you will present.

## Do Your Homework

It is important to research a Home before you go. Knowing the number of residents who live there, the space where you will perform, the types of disabilities represented and the percentage of residents with dementia are important factors. It also helps to note how many blind or deaf residents are there and the number of people who are heavily medicated.

You might want to ask if a PA system and tables are available so you know what you will have to take with you. The more information you gather before your visitation, the better prepared you will be to meet the needs and capabilities of your audience. The most valuable resource person can be the Recreational Director. This person knows the residents personally and can provide you with an overview of what to expect.

## The Basic Routine for All Homes

Allowing extra time is a must so that when I arrive I can unload my car, transfer my equipment and set it all up before the residents are expected to arrive in the designated area. I personally like to line up all of my props on a table, covering them with a lightweight colorful table cloth to conceal them.

Even though it is especially important to cover your props when presenting children's programs, I still like to add this suspense for the adults and seniors. Even they get caught up wondering: What is next? ☺

When entertaining a large group in a dining hall or activity area, the staff will gather the residents who eagerly await you.

Because I arrive early enough to be completely set up and ready to begin, this "resident entrance time" is a fantastic time for walking around to meet and greet. I shake hands with each resident while asking his or her name and, when I am telling the resident my name, I carefully and purposefully touch his or her shoulder or arm to make contact.

### Music and Smiles Are Universal

Because music and smiles are universal and ageless languages, I customarily begin and end my program with music and splatter tons of smiles throughout. Truthfully, many of your residents may not remember what they had for lunch that day, or even if they HAD lunch, but play "Amazing Grace" or "Jesus Loves Me" and they will smile and sing every word with you in their "Sweet, Sweet Spirit!"

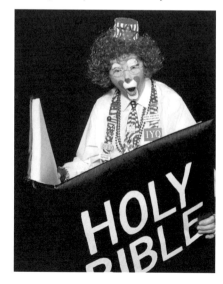

If I am going to residents with higher skills and more cognizant awareness, I make up large print sing along sheets for them.

I use Praise and Worship songs all year long and provide a Christmas sing-a-long booklet for this festive season. They love singing Christmas Carols. "Joy to the World, the Lord Is Come!"

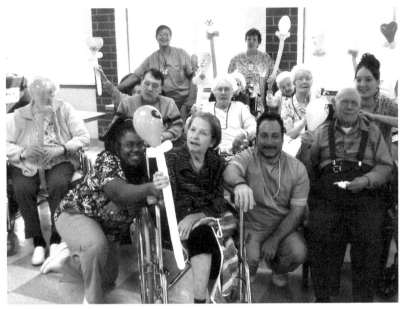

*Residents and staff of Seneca Place, Pittsburgh (above and next page) gather for a performance by Donna "Spangles" Shuster.*

While singing group songs, I always mingle among the flock shaking hands, touching shoulders, holding their hands and looking into their aged eyes. Those eyes always smile right back at you!

### Put Them in the Spotlight

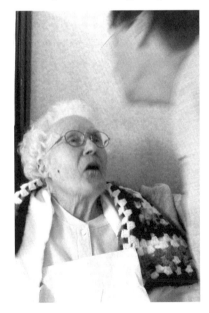

I find it so important and so much more fun to make the residents the center of attention. Put them in the spotlight! Give them a few minutes in the sun. Let the SON shine through them!

When I do my gospel clown magic, I use really big props, with a resident as my assistant. It is always the resident who makes the magic happen, not me. My chosen helpers

*Donna and her mother, Ruth "Granny" Reese, a resident of Seneca Place.*

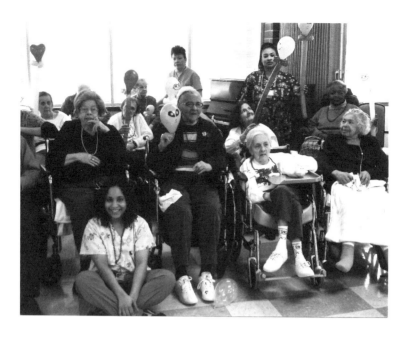

especially love it when their friends clap for them at the amazing feat they just performed. During my "meet and greet" time, I observe who appears to be alert, awake, and anxious for the program to begin. These people will be my assistants! Staff members can also specify which residents will make competent and congenial assistants. Use their wise counsel and recommendations as no one knows the residents better.

### The Amazing Blessing of Richard

Not too long ago, I had a blind man in my audience. He was loud, annoying and even a bit disruptive from my arrival until the beginning of my presentation. I could hardly wait to begin!

With silent prayers and an act of boldness, I decided to make Richard my first helper. He would either make or break me!

I was using my Blooming Bouquet bag. I had him feel the bag inside and out each time before HE produced the flowers. I had his friends describe the flowers he produced. He was intrigued by touching, feeling, measuring up, and trying to understand exactly what his friends could see. He was now getting all the attention without being a menace.

This was all he wanted—to be included! He was the most engaged, enthusiastic member of the audience for the remainder of our time together. (Thank you, Jesus!)

At the end of my program, I went around, held hands, said good-bye, put a red heart necklace around each one's neck, and reminded them: "God loves YOU!" When I got to Richard, I welled up as he clasped my hands in his saying, "Spangles, this is the very first time I ever SAW a magic show. Thank you!" He even invited me back the next day to have dinner with him.

What an awesome God we serve! No matter how many homes I visit, I always leave feeling that I personally am more blessed than when I arrived. God is faithful and true.

### Practice and Pray

I encourage you to step out of your comfort zone, practice, pray, practice and pray some more, and then go out there to serve these special people. They are hungry for your smiles, your touch, and your time with them. In fact, many of them are starving for your attention. Let us go together and serve them some spiritual food—serve them your special gifts in your own unique way.

### Room Visit Guidelines

It is extremely important to ask the nurses or aides if there are any residents whose rooms are "off-limits" to you. Often, the aides and activities staff will escort me to all of the rooms where they know I will be welcomed and enjoyed. When visiting rooms:

- Always knock, announce who you are, and ask permission to enter. Remember, you are entering their home!
- Speak loudly and slowly as you approach the resident. Greet them with your biggest smile and your warmest heart.
- Eye contact is vital.
- Many residents will not care if you are NOT in costume. They care mostly that YOU came to visit THEM.
- Just listening will be your greatest gift to them. Really HEAR what they are telling you and respond in a caring, appropriate manner.

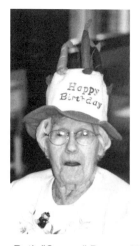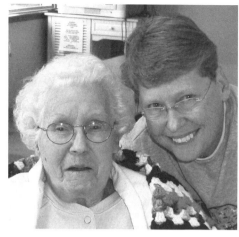

*Ruth "Granny" Reese, 95, with her daughter Donna "Spangles" Shuster*

- A little light story telling, a little pocket magic, a little song together, or just a little time—they will cherish your visit.
- Leave a bit of YOU behind. Without exception, I leave something with each resident to remind her or him of our special time together. Good choices are paper napkin roses, heart shaped beads (or any beads), or something that might be seasonal. I might add that ALL female residents LOVE their beads. They never have too many beads! Because I purchase my beads by the gross, they are not an expensive give-away and they provide joy for a very long time.

### Make a Difference

Nursing home clowning or just visiting makes a huge difference in the lives of many lonely, fragile people. Know ye this: Your visits with them will make a bigger difference in YOU, who you are, and why you do what you do.

We are privileged to have the gifts God gave us to be able to go into these homes. You will be truly blessed by blessing them with the sharing of your God-given gifts.

Again, what an awesome God we serve! Go ye therefore and step into this wondrous world of nursing home clowning!

God Bless YOU!

*Donna is president of Creative Artists for Jesus. To learn more about this organization and to contact Donna, see page 197.*

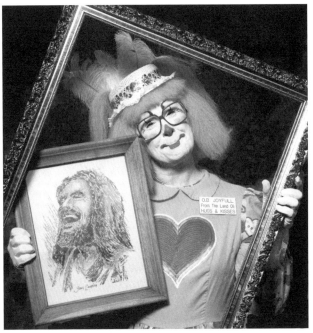

*Julie "O.B. Joyfull" Jahn with a picture of the "Laughing Jesus." by Ralph Kozak—see: www.jesuslaughing.com/*

### *Making of a Gospel Clown:*
# How "O.B. Joyfull" Came to Be

By Julie "O.B. Joyfull" Jahn

Hello, my name is Julie A. Jahn and I currently live on the east coast of the United States. I am your ordinary, average type American. I am divorced and remarried. Between us we have three children and seven grandchildren. I go to work; I eat; I sleep; I pray and I go to church. And when time allows, I volunteer. Strange as it may sound I even pay my taxes on or before April 15th of every year!

BORING, RIGHT? One day I was just minding my business doing ordinary boring things when everything changed. There in the mirror someone else was looking back at me. "Who was this person?" I asked. "Where did she come from?"

Let me back up a bit and start from the beginning. One day my current husband and I were wondering what to do. Stan (that's his name) and I had not been to the circus in a long time, so we thought, "Why don't we go to see the show in town. What a great idea!" We got tickets and away we went.

When we got to the circus, Stan said, "Why don't we have our faces painted up like clowns." (I would like to tell you that we had NO children with us, just him and me, and our combined ages at the time were close to 100 years old.)

### Then the Magic Began to Happen Inside of Me

So we had our faces painted and then the magic began to happen inside of me. The children who attended the circus were starting to run toward me.

"Miss Clown" they yelled and they gave me the biggest hugs. During the show the same thing happened. The children were coming to me in my seat asking me to do tricks, tell stories, do something funny. I was hooked! What a gift God gave me that day.

Well we went home and Stan said, "Julie why don't you find out where you can learn to be a clown." We looked and looked and all we could find was a clown school in Florida. (We lived in New Jersey then.) Florida was a little too far to travel everyday (big smile), so we put the idea on hold for awhile.

God was busy working behind the scenes and HE got me to meet some people, who knew some people, who knew some people that had gone to a local clown school. I got very excited and I called the magic store, signed up for the next class and met Fred Collins.

Fred's school was one night a week for six weeks. Fred taught us about clowning, make-up, juggling, skits, costumes, the ins and outs and the do's and do not's of clowning!

During this class an event called Clownfest was taking place along the New Jersey shore. Clowns from all over the U.S. and Puerto Rico came to learn, to compete and to be part of a HUGE Boardwalk Parade.

WOW! I was like a kid in a candy store. At the end of the four days of Clownfest, just before the BIG PARADE on the boardwalk, it happened again. The kids were running up to me—"Hey Miss

Clown" they yelled—giving me one hug after the other. I was hooked even more than before!

By this time I had my first costume and my first character that I called "Giggles." Well I was a new clown and did not know too much about the business. When I found out that some other person had the name trademarked, I had to change my name so I changed it to "Tickles." Well guess what? Someone else had that name too. I began to feel very sad. If just getting a name was this hard, then maybe I didn't really want to be a clown. But I was hooked so I had to do something.

I called a "seasoned" clown and we brainstormed for hours. After playing with many names and initials we finally arrived at "O.B. Joyfull." From then on there was no stopping me. I was hooked and I wanted to be the best I could be.

I learned how to do balloon sculptures, face painting and a little bit of magic. I started doing birthday parties, picnics, school presentations and more. Oh my! But I did not seem satisfied with this so I started talking to Jesus.

### Finding the Missing Piece: Clown Ministry

I thanked Him for this gift of O. B. Joyfull and I really was very happy, but something was missing. Jesus then led me to a Clown Ministry workshop.

"That's it—the missing piece," I said. "I want to be a Gospel Clown. I want to spread the Word of God, the joy, the laughter and the hugs of Jesus through the art of clowning."

Now I understood why God gave me the name O. B. Joyfull—from 2 Corinthians 5:17—"This means that anyone who belongs to Christ has become a new person. The old life is gone; a new life has begun!"

> I want to be a Gospel Clown. I want to spread the Word of God, the joy, the laughter and the hugs of Jesus through the art of clowning.

Oh how privileged, how honored, how proud I am to be commissioned by God Himself—that I am a new creation, given a new name, to go forth and spread HIS GOOD NEWS (Mark 16:15).

Over the past 15 years I have attended workshops, learned new skills, and worked on my makeup and costuming.

### See What God Has Done

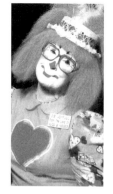

Many miracles have occurred in my life as a result of O. B. Joyfull. I have had the privilege of holding several offices in the World Clown Association including President for one year. I founded a group called Cheer Leaders for Christ, an organization that equipped and nurtured those in creative ministry. I have been fortunate to perform and teach in Canada and Europe. I wrote and produced a children's video called "Jesus Loves You." I have been gifted with several "clown friends" who are priceless.

My favorite things about clowning include:

- Making friends with that child or adult who was so afraid of "the clown" that they previously stayed away.
- Working one on one with a child or an adult.
- Visiting adult care centers and nursing homes.
- Teaching others to carry on the "art of clowning."

Julie "O. B. Joyfull" conducts workshops and retreats. She performs wherever the Lord sends her. She is God's servant under construction. My friend "Pete" always used to say to me, "Julie— learn something new every day and you will stay young."

I love learning new ways to present the gospel of Jesus Christ though joy, laughter and creative arts. I enjoy letting others laugh at me for being silly, so that through laughter they may forget their pain if only for a moment. What an honor and a privilege to be called personally by God to do this service (Colossians 1:25).

Through O. B. Joyfull, I am able to be child-like (NOT childish) in my relationship with the Lord. Praise Jesus! O. B. Joyfull is here to proclaim the Joy of the Lord. Won't you join me in remembering to be joyful unto the Lord always, again I say REJOICE (Philippians 4:4)!

*See Julie's routine on "Buckets of Love" on page 179. Visit her website at www.angelfire.com/planet/julieajahn  To contact her, see page 190.*

# Touch Them with God's Love

### By Pam "Sparky" Moody

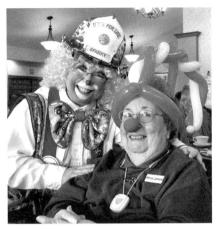

*"Sparky" with Wilma Lemons*

My character, Sparky, has been clowning in nursing homes since 1996. When I began with my clown ministry troupe, ACTS Clowns, we first started with a community room program. I quickly discovered that I most enjoyed working individually with residents.

Since my first real job in life was working in a nursing home at the age of 16, I developed an adoration and respect for the elderly. I also witnessed a great deal of loneliness and despair, as well as discovering how much first hand history could be learned simply by listening. I have found that the residents respond both to the humor shared as well as the brightly colored costumes.

One of my favorite gifts to share with the elderly is the gift of "touch." I have found that many residents yearn for a warm and loving touch and hugs are most always welcome.

I usually go with my "doggy bag" full of little walk around items, a bag of balloons and my giant kazoo ear (a giant plastic ear with a kazoo hot glued into it). This is because I don't read a bit of music, but I can sure play by EAR. I have found that most elderly residents have a favorite hymn and if they're lucky, I just might be able to hum a few bars. I usually have a few "red nose roses" on hand in case there is a special occasion.

Personally, I always try to work at eye level or below. I think it is much more respectful to residents to NOT be looking "down" on them as we talk or play. From personal family experience, I know to always get fairly close and keep direct eye contact. This enables residents with dementia to remain more focused and connected with what you're doing. If there is not a bed or chair

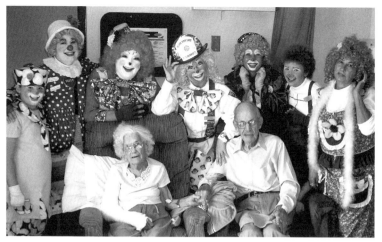

*Mr. and Mrs. Ray Runyon with (from left) Rachel "Hugs" Ramsey, Vicky "Trixy" Garrett, Norma "Harmony" Marvin, Pam "Sparky" Moody, Deb "Clickette" Cooper, Jennifer "Ida Know" Ramsey, Jan "Bubbles" Mosset*

nearby for me to sit, I usually will drop to one knee. I put kneepads under my costume for my own aging body!

One Sunday, after presenting a clown worship service in a small community, we dropped in on the nursing home before leaving town. One family summoned us to their parent's room. Their parents, in their upper 90's, had just been moved to the home the day before, after 70 plus years of marriage. They had lived independently before then and had a blessed life together.

The family was elated with our visit because it reinforced that this would be a FUN place for their parents to live. We took a group photo (above.) A few months later, I had the digital photo made into an 8 x10 print and returned to the home to deliver it. I found the husband in a different room alone. He shared with me that his wife had passed away only a couple of weeks after our visit. He was absolutely thrilled with my gift of a photo for his wall—the last photo of him and his wife together, holding hands surrounded by clowns. A memory he will always cherish.

Over the years, sharing in nursing home ministry has given me far more than I could ever give to anyone else. What a wonderful gift to share a giggle and a hug with such loving and receiving people. *Pam founded L.A.F.S. for Life. See more on page 195.*

# A Ministry of "Presence"

By Jan "Jaepers" Kerr

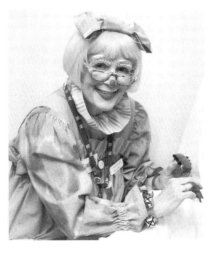

About 30 years ago, while away from home, I became very ill and required hospitalization. My family and friends did not know where I was, nor did I. With no one to visit me...no one to offer love and companionship...I relied upon the visits of a social worker and a chaplain to bring some measure of comfort to me. Of this experience, my mode of clowning was born.

Many persons ask if I "do" puppets, face painting, magic or storytelling. Well, yes I do, but my ministry to persons in eldercare facilities is more that of *presence* rather than of *props*. I am always there to listen and to provide a healing touch. I do, however, carry a small music box with me, allowing me an entree to those persons who do not yet know me or to those who are very ill.

One such person was Lily. She was well into her 80's. Seeing her in a state of illness and unable to converse because of several strokes caused former friends and family to limit their visits to her. Most of the time, her face was expressionless. But, over time, there was a faint hint of a smile when I came to visit her, and this small smile continued for each of my visits after that.

On my final visit to her, before she died, she reached up and cradled my face in her hand. Her eyes were filled with love. We understood each other. She understood that I loved her, and I understood that she also had come to love me.

God has given me a heart for persons who are lost, alone, and suffering. And bringing love and healing of spirit to these persons is my purpose. To God be the Glory!

*Jan leads The Merrimakers Clown Ministry at Aldersgate United Methodist Church in Wilmington, Delaware. To contact her, see page 191.*

# Be the Best You Can Be... and Then Get Better

## By Hal "Halaloo" Grant

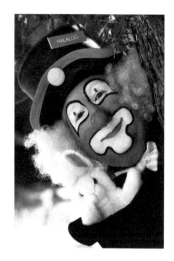

I have been clowning for a little over 10 years, primarily in Clown Ministry. Although nursing homes and assisted living facilities are not the main place I clown, I visit two or three care facilities a year.

If you are going to be a clown, be entertaining! Think of all the clowns who have come before you and those to follow: be the best clown you can be and then get better!

One of my favorite places to visit is where there are people with mental delays (all ages). We have a daughter with high needs who is delayed in all areas; she has taught me much about care clowning. Respect the space of all you meet, from room to wheelchair. For those in a wheelchair, the chair is an extension of their selves; respect that. Be gentle and play big. Ask permission before placing anything on the chair or tray.

### Entertaining Ways to Hand Out Gifts

I often am asked to hand things out—small gifts, stickers, beanie babies, etc. I always had a hard time thinking of how to do this and be funny or entertaining. The gifts may be in a bag—a Santa Sack works great at Christmas. It could be a wagon or service cart made into an Easter basket. If you can, dress it up.

You will also need a "change bag" (dress this up also) with a zipper! Have the person reach into the bag (non zipper side) and they find all sorts of things! Things I pretend I had lost. Next I reach into the zipper side (with zipper undone) and reach right through the bag and into the Santa Sack or onto the cart and pull the gift through the bag to give to those I am visiting. I sometimes use this as a way to reach into my pocket to pull out an effect to share. Play it up as much or as little as you feel is right.

*Visit Hal's website at* www.halaloo.com *To contact him, see page 189.*

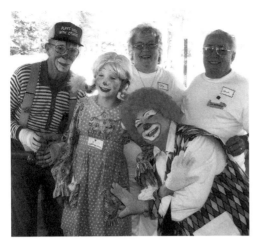
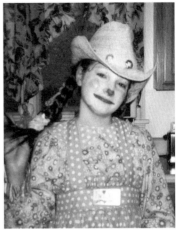

*From left, Jim "Pretzel" Cochran, Elizabeth "Twinkie" Cochran and Charlotte "Miz Frisbee" Cochran clown with their cousins. At right is "Twinkie."*

## What the Residents Love

By Charlotte "Miz Frisbee" Cochran

My husband Jim, who clowns as "Pretzel," and I have been visiting a nursing home once a month for the past five years.

We start by visiting room to room about 1 p.m. Then at 2 p.m. we go to a small activities room where 15 to 20 people are gathered. I take CD's for their CD player and we sing action songs such as "Tony Chestnut."

### *Favorite Songs*

Their most favorite song is "I like Friends" and they'll sing along with you—"*I like friends. I like you. I like to celebrate being a friend to you.*" (It is on The Learning Station: *Tony Chestnut and Fun Time Action Songs* CD.)

We take props for our songs. Jim takes an old baseball glove and a sponge ball for "Take Me Out to the Ballgame." We toss the ball to some of the men and they throw it back, or two of us as clowns toss it to one another. We use a thumb tip light for "This Little Light of Mine" and they like that.

We sing other favorite songs like "She'll Be Comin' Round the Mountain" and "Home on the Range." I'm 72 years old and if I know the songs I know they'll know them too.

Then we give out stickers which the residents love. They save them in special boxes in their rooms or in their Bibles.

Jim twists balloons and they love that. We make up the balloons in advance to save time there. We do short skits. We try

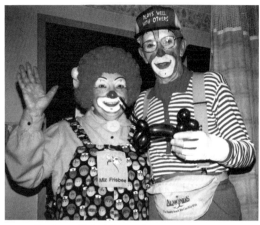

*Charlotte "Miz Frizbee" and Jim "Pretzel"*

everything out on them—all our new skits.

My granddaughter Elizabeth who often clowns with us as "Twinkie" has a puppet "Lamb Chop." The residents love puppets and stuffed animals. We're getting ready to do more with puppets.

### They Just Want You

But mostly what they want isn't even what you do. They just want you. They really just want a personal touch. They like to touch skin.

They look forward to our coming and the home puts it on its calendar. We don't visit during December because so many other visitors show up then but we always make it a point to visit in January and February because people don't visit then as much.

### An Amazing Breakthrough

Yesterday, a lady who always keeps her head down and never speaks, suddenly raised her head while we were singing "Jesus Loves Me" and she started to sing the words. I went over to her and I could understand her words.

It was the first time she had communicated in four years! Everyone was amazed. It made us all cry.

It showed me God is at work. It was an awesome thing.

*Charlotte and Jim Cochran, who also clown in hospitals, can be reached at 322 Williamson Rd., Greenville, PA 16125. See more on page 189.*

# Brighten Their Day

### By Rev. Bill Moore

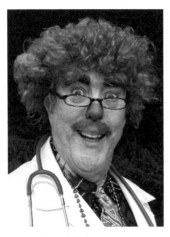

*Rev. Bill Moore as "DR Mal Praktiss"*

A clown brings attention to the resident and brightens their day. Even if a resident has cognitive difficulties, a clown can bring a smile. Some who rarely respond to outside stimuli will respond to the clown.

I always insist that someone from the activities department go with me to the residents' rooms because it offers a subtle reassurance to them that this funny looking character is okay. I stand back so the first person they see entering the room is someone they know. The staff person will say, "There's a clown here to visit you" or, "You have someone special here to see you."

Also, the staff person knows the residents. When I clowned in my other clown character—"Mo"—I would take my shy bear puppet with me. I would also take a tuba kazoo and ask them what their favorite song was. The two most requested songs were "You Are My Sunshine" and "Jingle Bells."

For some, just the memory and concept of a clown (for those who are cognizant) is a connection and the bright colors you wear delight the eye. As "DR Mal" I try to be very colorful. DR Mal doesn't sing or kazoo.

I think mornings are the best time to visit because the residents are more rested and alert than they are after a big meal. After lunch they usually take a nap.

My individual visits as DR Mal are short, so I can go to as many rooms as possible generating smiles. With those who are sharp, I will stay longer for some verbal bantering. What they don't need is someone to hang around. It's nice to lift them up but not tire them out. So many residents thank me for stopping by even for a one or two minute visit. To me it is a blessing to see them respond to the clown, so I get as much out of it as they do.

*Bill created the cartoons for this book. For more about Bill, see page 187.*

It brings a message
of joyful noise
and loving sounds
that takes them
to a place
perhaps long ago
—but for a few
minutes they
are "there again."

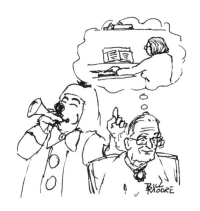

# The Ministry of Music

By Bobbi "Kizzy" Chard

My husband Dave and I have gone to nursing homes with a Banjo Band and the ministry of music is so rejuvenating and joyful to the people.

It brings a message of joyful noise and loving sounds that takes them to a place perhaps long ago—but for a few minutes they are "there again."

Music can be such a powerful ministry to all people. These people come up and thank us so profusely—one even came up and kissed my hand. It brought tears to my eyes.

Those residing in nursing homes are very special "saints" and they deserve all our love and care. The Lord has His Hands around these precious souls and we can do nothing short of taking this mission very seriously.

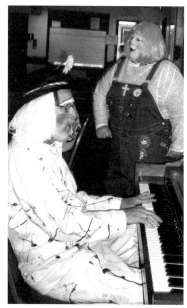

*Bobbi "Kizzy" Chard and Dave "Justy Nuff" Chard minister with music from banjos to pianos and singing.*

*To contact Bobbi and Dave, see page 188.*

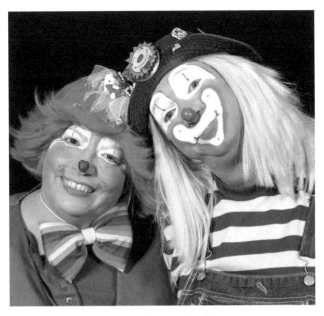

*Karen and Daniel Boudreaux*

# The Importance of Following the Spirit

### By Karen Boudreaux

I know a lot of new clowns go to nursing homes because the residents are a very forgiving audience. Honestly that is a fact. These people are so excited to have someone visit them that they are very loving and receptive. But just like with other audiences, you should ask God if there is anything in particular He wants you to do while there.

This rang true one time in our earlier days of clowning. There was one nursing home that the Grandma of my husband Dan was in. We loved this nursing home. It was clean and open and bright. The staff members were cheery and friendly and the residents were happier than at other homes we had visited.

There was one couple that unless the weather was really bad was always sitting on a swing on the front porch. It was really neat to see them sitting there holding hands. They always had a hello and a smile for us—even when we weren't "in clown."

---

Well one day we had two young girls who wanted to be clowns that came with us. They showed up late to our house and we had to make them up so we ended up running late for the performance. Because we were running late, we didn't notice that the sweet couple was missing from the porch.

Well the morning of the performance God had told me to do a song we didn't usually do "in clown." In the song the person was singing about how much he needed God through a heavy trial he was going through—that he knew no matter how hard the trial was, God would bring him through it one more time.

Well I had been to a few clown trainings and had read several books and was on all the clown lists and according to the lists this would not be an appropriate piece to do. It is not a depressing song but it is a very deep emotional piece.

So I prayed about it some more and I still felt very strongly to do it and so I did it. When we were done and packing up our stuff one of the staff came to get me.

There was the sweet little lady. One of the nurses had insisted she come to our "show." The poor thing was in tears and just wanted to hug me. She then told me how she had just lost her husband and didn't know if she would make it—until she saw us do that song. She thanked me and told me she just needed to be reminded. She squeezed my hand and said, "I can make it now."

## Another Time That God Led

As much as I love doing the shows at the homes, if at all possible I love going into the rooms of those that were unable to come to the show. Recently we were doing a show at a smaller home. There was a room right off of where we were doing the show. The man in the room was yelling and cursing throughout the whole show. The director kept apologizing for him and we kept on going trying to act like nothing unusual was happening. If he got especially loud we would stop for a minute and wait for him to quiet down and then go on. This wasn't a case of a heckler being in the room and I didn't know if this was normal behavior for him or if it was because he could hear us and all the laughter.

We went on with the show and then we visited with the people in the room. We packed up our props and told the director that we would like to visit some of the other residents. She started to direct us down a certain hall when I felt impressed to go see the old man that had been hollering. Now this wasn't a heroic gesture. I honestly was going because I felt impressed to do so.

The director asked if I was sure and told me that he could get very ugly. I swallowed and told her I was sure. Well as soon as I walked in the man started cursing up a storm. Instead of retreating I took a step closer. The man looked down and apologized. I told him, "That's okay." He then told me it was just that he hated his wife. He then started to call her some very ugly things. I just stood there and let him get it out. He then started telling me he hated her because she never came to see him.

Well, my mother had Alzheimer's. She was forever looking for my dad and asking me where he was. My dad had passed away a few years earlier but it didn't matter how much we told her she didn't remember. So I knew that there could be any number of reasons why this man's wife was not visiting him but there would also be a strong possibility that he wouldn't understand them.

So I just let him talk for awhile. He then looked me straight in the eye and told me, "I'm going to hell but I don't care because I hate that woman!"

Now I had not mentioned God or any of my beliefs but I can tell you I was silently praying and asking God what to say to this poor man. So when he told me he was going to hell and didn't care, that was my opening. I told him that I didn't believe that he didn't care if he went to hell or not.

He started yelling that all he cared about was that she had better go to hell for not coming to visit him. I told him I was sorry for what she had done but I couldn't do anything about that. I then told him again that he really didn't want to go to hell. He started crying. He told me no, he really didn't want to go to hell.

So I told him that he needed to forgive his wife. I told him that we aren't responsible for what others do but we are responsible for what we do. He told me he knew that and he was sorry for cursing at me. Later that day while we were visiting other patients, a nurse came up to me and said, "Honey I don't know what you told him but you can come back anytime. That is the most peaceful I've ever seen him."

A little forgiveness goes a long way. Sometimes these people in these homes don't need you to make them laugh. Sometimes they just need you to hold their hand or to just listen. That's why to me the most important thing in this type of clowning is to be led by the Holy Spirit.

*Karen and Dan's FreshFire Ministries involves drama, interpretive movement, dowel rod mime, clowning and flags. To contact them, see page 188.*

## Answering the Call

### By Luella Krieger

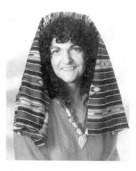

*Luella Krieger was a registered nurse for 21 years before receiving a call from God to serve Him full time in the ministry of drama and clown.*

I am rejoicing at the wonderful gift of clowning in those of you who are truly called and anointed to it. I remember once as I watched "Bubba" Sikes clown that I realized that some do clowning and some, like "Bubba," are anointed in it. You all have a high call from above.

I praise God for giving me the vehicle of clown to learn where my true calling is—that of storytelling. In two years my "Whinny the Klown" will retire but the lessons learned in magic and loving will live on in the storytelling character who will come after her.

As to nursing home clowning, I look back on my career in nursing, especially the years in nursing home administration, and know that those who are called to clown in that setting are above and beyond anointed. It is one thing to be called and another to answer the call.

Thank you all for answering.

*Visit Luella's ministry at www.fool4christ.org/ To contact her, see page 193.*

# Cooking Up Fun

## By Karen "Tickitty Boo" Oke

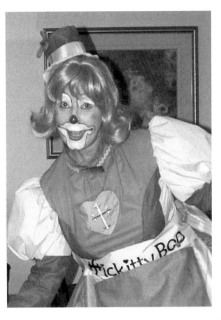

I've found seniors enjoy two routines with everyday kitchen items. The first routine is better for those whose minds can still grasp puns. To start the first one, I've used a plastic *A&P grocery store bag.* I ask, "Does the A&P stand for Adoration and Praise? No? Sorry, I must have been mistaken."

I take out of the bag a can of *brown beans* and say, "Once I was just an average human bean. Life was okay and I made all my own decisions until I got into a real *pickle.* I didn't know where to turn. I started to pray and watch (*Spray and Wash*) and finally I gave my *LIFE* (cereal) to Christ.

"Now things aren't always perfect. I have a lot of bittersweet (*chocolate*) situations but I always remember that God is in control (*pantyhose*). He has made me glad"(*Glad garbage bags*). I usually finish with a bag of slivered *almonds* and say, "Amen!"

### Hot Cookies

I keep my eyes and ears open to everything that I MIGHT be able to develop into a clowning routine. This I developed from a devotional contributed by Judy Miller, Alberta Canada, on the Presbyterian Church in Canada's Daily Devotional website, <daily.presbycan.ca> She gave me permission to adapt it into a clown skit.

I plunk on a chef's hat and two of the dollar-store oven mitts and reminisce about being a kid waiting for the hot cookies to come out of the oven. If I took them out too early, they would be raw and not ready. If I didn't let mom turn it to the correct temperature, the ingredients didn't go through the necessary process. I had to wait even longer when they came out or my tongue would burn.

Our Christian experience is a long one, period. We want to change in the blink of the eye, but we need patience. We don't want the hot seat and trials that come but we need to have the ingredients in our life go through this process. Then I thank them for being patient with me and my silliness. I thank them for being kind and attentive. It's a great note to end on.

*To contact Karen, see page 195.*

# Adapting Skits with Your Creativity

Karen Oke's grocery store skit shows the creative adaptations one can make. She credits her original sourcing to both Hal "Halaloo" Grant (page 121) and Carol "Blossom" Kay (page 96.)

Hal created a shopping list testimony 8 to 9 years ago with products found in Canada. He calls his skit "Shopping for Mom."

Carol's skit, "Testimony by Groceries," dates to the early 1990's. She also uses Canadian products. She adapted her idea from Randy Christensen's "Testimony Food" in Janet Litherland's *Everything New and Who's Who in Clown Ministry* (1993).

### Add a Christian Message to Your Skit

Consider adapting skits such as "Ring Ring" (page 168) with a Christian message. Have the other clown say, "Can you hear me? Can you hear me now?" Then ask, "What are you trying to do?"

They say, "I'm trying to call God." Then you say, "That's not how you do you it. You need a special phone." And then do the regular Ring Ring. After they pull the trick on you say, "You got me on that. Isn't it good that God never plays tricks. We don't really need a special phone to call God. God hears our prayers and His line is never busy. He always answers."

### A Good Christian Skit Book

*To God Be the Glory! A book of Christian Ministry Skits, Magic and Miscellaneous Items* by Barry DeChant is available for $7 plus postage from Barry DeChant at 4215 64th Avenue East, Sarasota, FL 34243. Telephone: (941) 351-6572. Email: bonzkari@aol.com

To GOD be the Glory!

A book of Clown Ministry Skits, Magic, and Miscellaneous Items

by Barry DeChant

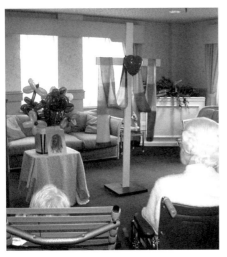
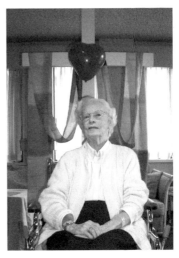

*Large visuals are easily seen such as the rainbow scarf draped over a cross with a large heart balloon or balloon flower bouquets. At top right, Laura Gionesto sits "beneath the cross" after services at The Fairways at Brookline.*

## Lead Worship with Bright Visuals

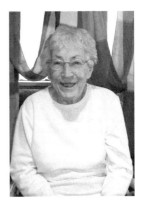

Use your skills as a clown to make balloon animals such as a Lion (below) to tell the story of Daniel in the Lion's Den.

Give residents pictures of themselves in their "Sunday Best" as shown by Martha Weaver sitting beneath the cross at right.

Residents love to sing familiar hymns. Give them large-print words on sheets as held by Wilma Hosterman below right. For more worship ideas, see page 149.

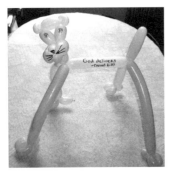
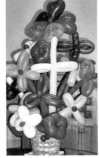
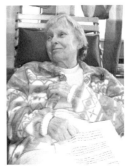

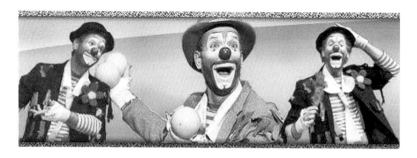

# The Art of Clowning

By Rev. Randy Christensen

Clowning can be an art. It's not automatically an art but it may become an art. Just because a person plays with play dough does not mean he is an artistic sculptor. Because a lady can jump in the air does not mean she is a prima ballerina. And just because a person slaps on make-up and has had a few classes does not mean that he has become a clown artist.

As I spent time in prayer, I believe God spoke to my heart about "art." Art is simply and purely the creative expression of the soul. Mark 12:30 states we love the Lord with all of our heart and soul..." and verse 31 says, "Love your neighbor as yourself..." We use artistic expression to show our love to God, and also to share our hearts and soul with others.

God loves seeing us express ourselves through art. Consider His own wonderful artistic creation in this galaxy.

So, how does clowning move to the level of "art" rather than simply "play?" To become an artist requires a long-term time investment to develop the disciplines of the art form. Artistry often is developed under the direction of a master. Artistry only accelerates as the person becomes focused on improving small specific details to ensure a successful product.

Clown from your heart and present your very best. Offer the love of God from your soul to your audience. You too can bring a wonderful experience to people as you share the art of clowning.

*Reprinted with permission from* www.pastorclown.blogspot.com/
*Visit Randy's website* www.randysinfo.com/ *for clown ministry books and resources. For more on Randy's ministry and to contact him, see page 189.*

---

# Chapter 8
## Clowning in Alzheimer's Units

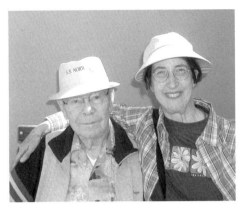

*My beloved step-dad, Paul Gosney, once quipped upon seeing me, "Ah, a familiar face." Though Alzheimer's has impaired much of his memory, his sweet character remains. Here we're pictured in the garden area at his Florida facility.—Anita Thies*

When I prepare to visit an Alzheimer's unit, I think of an adaptation of Simon and Garfunkel's song *Feelin' Groovy:* "Slow down, you move too fast. You gotta make the 'moment' last."

I'm so aware from my own relatives who have dementia that the moment is all they have. Not the future. And less and less of the past. The challenge is to make a positive connection with them in their moment. In this chapter, Elizabeth Plozner, Korey Thompson and Karen Baxter discuss ways to do that.

### When You Are Asked to Entertain

There may be times when you are asked to entertain at community room programs with family present. For such occasions, I've found the residents like colorful props that relate to familiar songs and experiences of days gone by.

Producing the rainbow scarf (see page 185) for "Somewhere Over the Rainbow" taps into memories. One time a resident spontaneously sang all the words and wound up doing a duet with the Judy Garland recording. The other residents loved it. They also like to sing "Take Me Out to the Ballgame."

In a recent program, residents loved seeing the clowns' big shoes. When a clown did the "Growing Taller" skit (see page 167) one of the residents volunteered the punch line before it came. Routines such as the Round Balloon Blowup (page 174) do well.

These allow residents to watch the antics of a clown without having to process spoken language. Remember that their cognitive challenges increase the time they need to take in what you're doing.

Many times, you can involve family members as your helpers. Bringing laughter to the family is a welcome respite for them. Making balloon animals provides a shared, lighter moment as do wearing clown noses, playing kazoos or giving them hand shakers to keep time to the music.

## How Clowns Can Be a Connecting Force

By Elizabeth Plozner

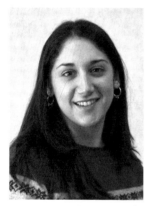

As the activities director at The Terrace at Brookline, my job is to give our residents inspiration and motivation —mentally, physically, and emotionally. Even though they have dementia, they never lose the need to be stimulated and emotionally connected with those they love and are surrounded by.

The reason we bring in clowns or any entertainment is because family members of residents feel they've lost connection with their loved ones. Clowns can be a connecting force.

We bring in entertainment monthly to connect families as, together, they watch a clown or celebrate the holidays. Family members also bring their children. We try to make the entertainment appropriate for all ages. It gives the families a chance to see their loved ones in different ways. With sing alongs, for instance, some families may not have heard their resident sing for a very long time.

The most important thing is to make it lighthearted and fun and enjoyable. The clown assists in our mission by helping residents feel positive emotions. They say it only takes 17 muscles to smile compared to 44 muscles to frown. To see someone laugh is the best part of my day. Many people have the misconception that residents are sleepy and express no emotion but I find that isn't true.

## When You Clown

When you clown, use visual humor and a change of tone in your voice to indicate that something is funny. Use emotional facial expressions, use your hands and use body language to help communicate. Everyone picks up on body language.

Tactiles are very important—clown noses, kazoos, balloon animals. When residents see and touch them, their brains are stimulated to a different level.

In your entertaining, work with associations. For instance, say, "What reminds you of February? Valentine's Day? Chocolate? Boyfriends? Flowers." It's all about getting the brain to work and trying to remember things.

You could say, "How many of you like football?" or, "What did you see at a circus?" It's incorporating them into the experience of your entertainment.

Sing-alongs are a great way to end your programs any time of day. I've heard that the last part of memory to go is music. It's amazing to watch them sing. An excellent way to close is with the song "You are My Sunshine."

## One-on-One Visits

For one-on-one visits, on your first visit, go around with the activity director who will help you get acquainted and will tell you whether to call them Mr. or Mrs. or by their first name.

The activity director can also tell you something special about them. There's always a good quality and a fascinating history about everyone.

The residents know my face and my voice even though they may not remember my name. They will come to recognize you as a friendly face. So put on your friendly face and let them know you're here for them.

You can introduce yourself and say, "I'm happy to be here and I'm happy to see you." If they don't know their own name, you could say, "I could call you Miss Blue Eyes." Say something that will encourage them and make them smile without treating them childishly.

You want to make them feel special and compliment them e.g., "Aren't your blue eyes beautiful." It shows you are aware of them and that they have worth.

Obviously you don't want to "dumb down." Many residents were prominent professionals and you don't want to be calling them "sweetie." And you don't want to put them on the spot.

When you approach, if they look away or walk away or get hesitant, it is best to casually wave to them but don't approach them. Once they see that others are friendly to you, they might warm up to you.

Regarding touch—you can gently graze their shoulder. The most important thing is that you have that connection that says, "I'm here for you."

If you don't get eye contact by a casual graze at the shoulder, then gently caress their hand and say, "I'm ____ the clown and I'm going to be the entertainer today."

### The Best Time to Visit

The best time to visit is mid-morning and afternoon. Evenings can be the worst because some residents experience what is known as "sun downing." Sun downing doesn't happen to everyone. It's a time when they are more frazzled and agitated. They are trying to hold onto every last memory and the sense of themselves is not there. So if you do clown in the evenings, it's best to do more singing.

### Lasting Rewards

Even though they may not remember what you said or did, you will remember that you gave them joy in the moment and that their family members saw them happy. What better reward could there be for a clown or any entertainer?

*Elizabeth Plozner is Activities Director at The Terrace at Brookline, 610 West Whitehall Rd., State College, PA. 16801. She holds a degree in Human Development and Family Studies from The Pennsylvania State University with a specialization in Advanced Aging and Development.*

# Hearts Open to Possibility Each Day (HOPE)

### By Karen "Rootin' Tootin' Newton" Baxter

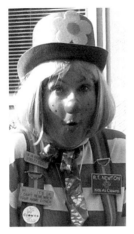

In my years as both Therapeutic Clown and HOPE KID Facilitator with Capital Care Strathcona in Sherwood Park, Alberta, Canada, I have come to recognize that feelings of confusion and panic dwell in the minds of most of the Alzheimer residents I've encountered.

Recently, I asked Anna, a resident with Alzheimer's, what she'd like to do? Her agitation was immediately apparent, in the flare of a nare, and the shrill in her voice!

"How would I know?" she cried. "I'm just an old lady. I don't know what I want to do! Tell me what to do, and I'll do it."

I was momentarily taken aback, but quickly responded, "Let's watch TV. Perhaps you will enjoy that."

"I hope so," Anna replied.

I hope so too, I thought, for it saddened me to think that perhaps Anna hadn't enjoyed herself for a very long time.

My initial response to Anna's reaction was embarrassment. I was embarrassed because Anna had reprimanded me. I had missed her cues of frustration and helplessness. The signs were there. In fact, in our bi-weekly encounters, they had rarely strayed. It didn't matter what activity the HOPE KIDS engaged the residents in, Anna's confusion was apparent. Bewilderment cloaked her like a felonious fog. She never knew what to do, or where to go. When she was directed to a spot, her eyes momentarily searched for some glimmer of familiarity regarding her surrounding, and the strangers in it. Flustered, she would demand, "What am I doing? I don't know what to do."

At times, I have been immersed in my own fog of confusion in relating to the "Annas" at the Care Centre. I have no iron-clad strategy for alleviating their confusion or panic, or the effects that meds have on their already muddled minds.

On "good" days, for a brief time, if we're lucky, we help Alzheimer residents enjoy a meaningful moment. It is often a mutual construction, with resident and HOPE KID* or resident and Clown interacting together. It is a moment of connection, a hopeful encounter, where sunshine occludes the cloud of anxiety.

We cannot always identify the key that unlocks the "moment." It could be a hug, a game, a picture, an aroma, a song, a joke, a story, a greeting, a cup of tea, or a smile.

It is enough to know that when we beckon with kindness, hearts open with possibility, enabling one human being to connect with another, if just for a moment.

Perhaps this poem I wrote, inspired by my encounters, will express what I feel to be true in sharing HOPE with Alzheimer residents if they could share their perspective:

> Just for this moment
> You are my mother's voice
> Gently caressing my soul
> With your tender touch
> Of reassurance.
>
> Just for this moment
> You are my daughter's voice
> Giggling and laughing
> Splashing me with
> Your shower of rainbows.
>
> Just for this moment
> You are my sister's voice
> Chiding and teasing
> Beckoning and calling me
> To play hide and peek with you.
>
> Just for this moment
> You are a clown's voice
> Reacquainting my heart
> With the warm glow of friendship
> And making me smile.

*For more on the HOPE KIDS, see page 161. For Karen's Nursing Home humour ideas see page 106. To contact Karen, see page 188.*

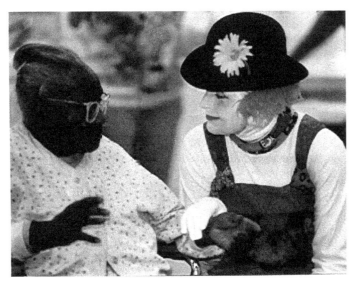

*Korey "Tunkal" Thompson with an Alzheimer's resident*

### *To Dance with Their Spirit:*
# Will You Wait for Them?

## By Korey Thompson

Clowns engage the dance of our spirit. Regardless of the venue, feeling safe and loved is an invitation for our spirit to come out to play.

Whenever someone inquires about clowning with Alzheimer's patients, my first question is, "What draws you to clowning with people who have dementia?"

Clowning in any therapeutic setting is a specialized field. It's not focused on the clown's traditional tricks or snappy appearance. It's all about the person you meet and whatever *their* needs are. In this venue the clown must be flexible in clowning style and willing to not take themselves too seriously.

The essence of clowning with dementia patients is the same as any kind of effective interpersonal interaction. A good clown helps set the stage through proper pacing, a playful attitude and visual stimulation. I will suggest some ways to tailor these elements to dementia work (play) later in this article.

## The Personal Challenge

Perhaps the most challenging part of clowning with dementia patients comes when the clown's own unresolved personal issues are unexpectedly triggered by a patient's illness or condition. For instance, we might see hints of our own aging face in the person in front of us and tremble at the thought. Or we might be reminded of a loved one who faced similar challenges in the past. Once those images capture our attention, the person in front of us falls to second place behind our own personal drama! At the very least, the authenticity of the present moment is at risk.

If we truly wish to serve others, their needs must come before our own. Being compassionately honest about old hurts or unfinished business might have us postpone this type of work until greater personal peace unfolds.

## The First Visit and Return Visits

When an agreement for making clown visits is established between you and a care giving facility, it's wise to consider making the first visit in street clothes, not in costume. In addition to meeting some of the residents and getting a feel for the pace of activities, this visit provides an ideal opportunity to begin building a relationship with staff. Staff people are your best allies, cueing you with names of people to visit, suggestions on levels of activity that are appropriate and much more. As you and the staff get to know and trust one another, a subtle nod of the head or a half sentence introduction can be invaluable.

The preliminary visit to the facility also acquaints you with the layout of the building and helps you identify possible locations for interaction. Later when you make your first visit in clown persona, you'll be less anxious and better equipped to concentrate on the real reason you're there.

## Potential Stumbling Blocks

As visits progress and relationships develop between clown and patient, you may fall victim to a couple of assumptions which are distinctly unhelpful in dementia work. One is that a previous meaningful encounter will carry over to the next encounter with that person. Even though I may fondly remember a meaningful interaction from one meeting, the next time I see that person I may be regarded as a total stranger at best or a complete nuisance at worst. Thankfully, there are many times when memory serves well and that's great. But be prepared to start at Square One again every time.

Another potential stumbling block is assuming that a person who is typically friendly or compliant (or vice versa) will continue to act in the same manner as time goes by. The disease process of dementia can include phases of great agitation, hostility, or detachment. Those phases may be brief or lengthy.

Common assumptions about the way human relationships typically go don't always serve us well in this setting. In dementia work, *all we have is the moment.* And in all honesty, isn't that about the way life is anyway?

### Be Prepared and Also Wide Open

Clowning in a therapeutic setting calls for being extremely well prepared and wide open at the same time. The preparation is really a form of hospitality which helps the patient feel comfortable and honored. The wide-open part is being willing to engage and enjoy a moment of play at an appropriate level.

Dementia has some unique characteristics. For example, even when <u>cognitive</u> processes become compromised, <u>emotional</u> processes may be fairly intact or at least diminishing at a slower rate. This means that even if the patient's understanding or speaking of words is bollixed up, body language still speaks loud and clear. If you're feeling nervous or in a hurry, that will be understood contrary to anything you might say. So keep it real! It's an honorable way of relating to others.

Hospitality also includes the process of creating a physical environment which is conducive to meaningful interaction. Comfortable lighting and temperature and a place sheltered from excess noise or people hurrying by is more pleasant for everyone.

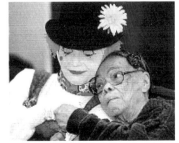

Patients will signal if a situation is upsetting or if they're uncomfortable in some way. The most common signals are distraction, shutting down, or exhibiting aggressive behavior. It's equally important to remember that the dementia patient may just not feel like playing some days—a very human choice to make. They get to choose, and we get to hear the message with grace and not take it as a personal affront.

## Waiting 90 Seconds Without Anxiety

Medical research in dementia indicates it can take up to 90 seconds for the brain with dementia to process a question or an instruction. In our sound-byte culture, a minute and a half is a long time to wait for a response. The temptation is to repeat the question or instruction in the meanwhile and perhaps with increased volume. Unfortunately this only tends to restart the 90 second clock again and the heightened volume or urgency of the request becomes part of the message too.

So a clown needs to know how to wait with grace and without anxiety. Kick back into a relaxed but "attentive" pace while you wait. Sometimes I will cock my head gently to the side (a non-confrontational pose) and quietly hum to the music or say "Ummmmm. . ." in a way that is not intrusive. When folks perceive you're staying with them in their space and at their pace, a meaningful response is more likely.

## Eye Contact: Be Shy and Woo Them

A good way is to make eye contact from a distance as you approach. Give patients an opportunity to look you over from a safe distance and then *smile* as you make brief eye contact, perhaps three seconds or so. Your body should be angled just a bit to one side rather than a full-frontal stance which is a universal symbol of power or confrontation. Look down and to the side after you've made the first eye contact—then look up and *smile* and make eye contact again. It's helpful if you look away before they do, at least part of the time.

Next time you look up you could wave gently and see if they will wave back. If they do, mirror the breadth and speed of their wave—you're already starting to pace their level of comfort.

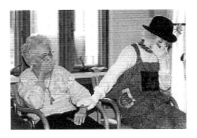

Woo them—maybe put your hand to your mouth one time and act shy like you're not quite sure how to take the next step in making contact. Allow them the space to take initiative.

Taking a few steps forward and then *pausing* is a way of inviting them to the interaction. Don't rush. Even if they recognize you from before, allow time for them to get onboard with the idea that you're here again.

When you get that distinct "Aack!" look in any situation, gently wave goodbye, smoothly turn away and obviously direct your attention elsewhere so they do not feel it's necessary to protect their space. This is not a conquest of wills and they well may choose to engage you later.

It's a good idea to keep body language consistent with your message. For instance don't be holding some interesting-looking colorful prop in your hand when you're trying to establish eye contact. Take one thing at a time and establish a connection with them first. The rest can unfold as an exchange between friends.

### Let Them Be Part of the Gag

Humor can act as an important expression of respect and belonging. Clown gags typically work by resolving some concocted problem with an unexpected resolution. When we as observers "get it" we not only delight in the surprise of the absurd answer, we become part of a group who is in the know.

Practicing humor in an appropriate way shows respectful regard to those with dementia. To help make humor accessible, replace clever spoken jokes with visual/sight gags. Cueing appropriate times for laughter can help include everyone in the elite group who gets it.

There are at least two major benefits of using humor in dementia care. First, studies show that just laughing for laughing sake delivers benefits to body and spirit. The successful cognitive process of mentally getting the joke is gravy. Secondly, the process of sharing a laugh is an elemental expression of connection. Dementia is a highly isolating condition and participating in an experience of connection provides an experience of context and community.

The laughing mirror is often a good prop—look into the mirror and the mirror laughs back at you. The sound of the canned laughter often elicits a laugh in return.

A juicily "bad" prop is the fart machine. Everybody does the socially impolite deed, making it ideal for safe but slightly rebellious humor. Depending on the level of functioning of the person, sometimes I push the button or push it the first time and then invite the patient to push it. I usually hold the machine in my hand to guide the timing. This helps guide the situation to lean toward success and not failure. If someone is genuinely offended by the gag, you can simply say, "Oh my goodness!" and just put the box away as if you were embarrassed or shocked by it yourself.

Staff can be great straight-men/women in this gag as well. Pushing the button as staff walks by and then wildly fanning the air usually gets a laugh. Staff frequently are more than willing to play along and the resident can get quite a kick out of putting the potty humor on someone else.

### Another Version of the Dance

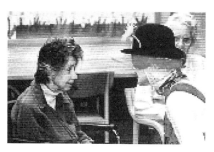 One of my all-time favorite activities in dementia work is dancing with people while they are seated in a chair. With music playing and my body just slightly angled to signal non-aggression, I approach with my palms up. As I do so I imagine the softest, most precious thing I can think of in my hands.

Almost without fail the person will place their hands on mine so our hands are together palm-to-palm and we can gently sway to the beat of the music. _At least_ half the magic depends on them. You can see it in their eyes!  It's great.

## Some Tips that Have Worked for Me

- If you enter someone's space and things go badly, you can leave the room and try again in about 5-10 minutes. Let memory loss work in your favor!

- I like to use music when working with dementia patients. People usually find it relaxing and it bridges the quiet times in communication. Choice of music is vital and I definitely recommend assembling your own mix of music. If you enjoy the music, chances are your pleasure and comfort will be communicated.

- Aim for music with a steady pulse and a generally upbeat mood. Avoid weepy songs or my-brother-shot-my-dog themes, or songs with sudden, fast passages or long quiet periods. Avoid dissonant harmonies. Men especially seem to like an occasional Sousa march, but watch the tempos.

- Music with about 70 beats per minute is a good choice. That pace approximates the rate of the human heart.

- Check out folk music from many parts of the world. You'll often find simple melodies with pleasing harmonies. A familiar tune now and again can be fun to hum or sing along with.

- I use a clown cart to carry my music player and maybe a few props. Transporting props in the box is risky because some folks just love unloading colorful items and hurry them off to points unknown when you're otherwise occupied. Carrying a few props in pockets works better.

- Small items like clown erasers are inappropriate because of the likelihood that they will be eaten.

   Remember your venue regarding makeup: use a light touch and avoid expressions that could be interpreted as anger or hostility. Proportions for up-and-personal interactions should be much smaller than for a parade where you want to be seen from a distance.

- Always allow patients to say "no" to a clown visit even if you have your heart set on it. Remember it's always about them and not about us.

- If you have a moment of encountering a mannerism or situation that repulses you at some level but is not harmful to the patient, focus *DIRECTLY ON THEIR EYES.* Look beyond whatever upsets you and <u>look into their eyes</u>. What you're apt to see there is likely to melt any fear or disdain.

- If you encounter a situation where a patient could be at risk, report that to a staff person and let them handle it. Also don't offer food, candy or drink to a patient, or help a patient get out of bed, etc. Let the staff handle their part of the bargain.

Sometimes when I share stories about working with people with dementia some mistakenly assume that it's one poignant interchange after another. Oh, wrong! Even though this kind of clowning reminds me of one of the reasons I'm on the planet, it's still the common grit of life—a blend of comic casualties and good days all wrapped up in one.

### Why I Love Clowning with Dementia Patients

Appreciation of elders is part of my family tradition. My Dad in particular always made sure that we kept in touch with family which resulted in an ongoing series of weekend visits to aging relatives. Over and over I got to witness people who had "gotten a little funny" in their old age start acting more like themselves

and genuinely enjoying the company.

Although I never would have expressed it this way at the time, I learned to trust the healing power of caring and human contact.

Clowns can bring a bit of color and novelty to mundane tasks, and that's a breath of fresh air. When a clown first plans to be regularly involved in a care giving situation, it's important to seek some kind of training. Training in clown techniques, understanding some basic characteristics of dementia, and the care giving protocols at the site can improve the odds of making a connection and lessen frustration for everyone involved.

As life comes to a close in the final stages of dementia, the flicker of the patient's spirit is surely more illusive. The conventional techniques of making a connection become far too cumbersome. It's heart to heart at this point.

One way to think of visits then might be to compare it to an impromptu visit to a friend in regular life only to find out they're not home right then. Perhaps you'd leave a little note telling them you stopped by and wishing them well.

So if no one happens to "be home" when you visit, a way of letting the person know you stopped by might be to pause to touch their hand and share a few quiet words with them. Maybe you remember aloud or in your heart a special time you shared with them. In other words, you affirm each other's spirit just like you've always done.

Clowns don't show up to *fix* anything. They come to dance in the face of life as it is, and when that happens we know we're not alone on this journey. And that is sufficient.

*For more on Korey, see page 199.*

## Resources from Korey Thompson

Korey Thompson has produced two videos of her work with dementia patients. These videos demonstrate the pace of the interaction and how to identify and interpret the fleeting cues of this intuitive work. Although the work is subtle, cues are there if you know what to look for.

The first video (approx 16 min, $35 +S/H), "Introduction to Therapeutic Clowning," is an introduction to clowning in a therapeutic situation. The second video (approx 21 min, $50 +S/H), "Making the Connection," outlines specific steps of creating a safe place and making interpersonal connections. This video also shows how to identify and respond to the hesitation that so often occurs in making a connection when you're not sure about whether to proceed or end the encounter. The pair of videos run $70 + S&H.

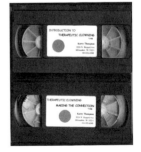

See Korey's updated email and postal addresses on this book's website at www.angelfire.com/planet/nursinghomeclowning

## Resources from the Calvin Institute of Christian Worship

There are wonderful resources that may be downloaded for free from http://www.calvin.edu/worship or you may contact the Calvin Institute of Christian Worship—Calvin College, 1855 Knollcrest Circle SE, Grand Rapids, MI 49546-4402 (616) 526-6088 for free or low cost resources.

The Institute's materials includes a pilot worship and activity program that was created for higher-functioning people with dementia at Holland Home in Grand Rapids, Michigan. Materials also include a booklet of "Prayers and Rituals of Blessings for Our Later Years."

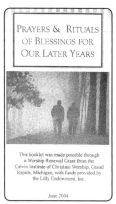

The article excerpted below was first published by the Calvin Institute of Christian Worship, http://www.calvin.edu/worship/ (Reprinted with permission.)

At Holland Home in Grand Rapids, Michigan, the Evening Star committee spent an intense six months of learning before they began to write and test their worship and activity curriculum. They consulted dementia, education, and interactive music experts; sponsored a conference on dementia and worship, and visited Montessori classes.

"With dementia people, the last thing into the brain—speech, intricate thinking—is the first thing out. They slowly regress to childhood. You can't teach anything new. Instead you have to touch and revisit what they already know," says Phil Lucasse, a Holland Home board member and retired college education professor.

It's heartbreaking to watch age or dementia claim a loved one's mind, body, and spirit. But it's a mistake to think that disease destroys a Christian's desire or ability to worship. Older adults can still encounter God through well-designed worship services.

Among their recommendations are to:

- Speak slowly, use large gestures, and pause for recognition time.
- Use familiar sensory cues to prompt holy remembrance and encourage faith-filled responses.
- Use props that people can see and touch, such as a cross, Bible, and communion table elements.
- Choose classic songs, such as "What a Friend We Have in Jesus," "Amazing Grace," and "Abide with Me."
- Consider using a Bible story picture book to tell the story.
- Babies first know love through touch and their parents' loving glances. Instead of giving a general blessing, make it personal. Touch each worshiper and look right into his or her face.

# Chapter 9: Be Santa and Mrs. Claus

Who better to bring the "Ho Ho Ho" of happy memories than those with clown skills? As you read these testimonials by Carole "Pookie" Johnson and Ruth "Angell" Matteson, I hope you will consider adding a Santa or Mrs. Claus persona (and their wonderful wardrobe) to your outreach.

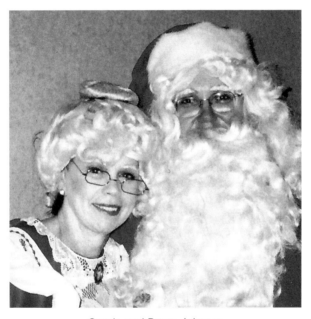

*Carole and Bruce Johnson*

## See Their Eyes Light Up

By Carole "Pookie" Johnson

For my husband Bruce and me, a highlight of our holiday season is volunteering in area nursing homes as Santa and the lovely Mrs. Claus. Nursing home residents may forget many things, but they never forget Santa! (And few have ever even seen Mrs. Claus in their whole life!)

The women in particular are fascinated by my red velvet dress and white lace apron.

> **Nursing home residents may forget many things but they never forget Santa!**

I let ladies feel how soft the fabric is. Sometimes this leads into a discussion about sewing.

## *Our Greatest Reward*

To see their eyes light up is our greatest reward. Bruce is a wonderful Santa and we both, without even really realizing it, use our clown skills in our interactions.

We have a favorite joke where Santa asks me, "Did you see the snow, Honey?" I reply, "No, but I saw the rain, dear." Remember, we are from Seattle.)

Sometimes a nursing home asks if we will come and hand out Christmas presents to the residents. We prefer not to do this. We think people who know the residents can distribute the gifts more efficiently. It is better to use our talents interacting with the residents and staff.

We take candy canes with us. We don't give any to the residents because we don't know what diet restrictions they have. We give them to the staff as a way to say thank you to them. Sometimes we have gone to entertain at the Staff Christmas Party.

## *Pictures to Treasure*

One of the things that we do as Santa and Mrs. Claus is posing for photos with the residents. The nursing home supplies its own camera. We can't use our camera because of the HIPAA law (Health Insurance Portability and Accountability Act) which protects resident's privacy. The nursing homes like the photos because they are proof for relatives of the residents that the home is having activities.

We have had some wonderful pictures taken of us with three or four generations of a family visiting for the party. Last Christmas a woman sat next to Santa. Her daughter and granddaughter stood behind them. Her great granddaughter sat on Santa's lap. What a picture for them to treasure!

After the party we enjoy going room to room to visit those who were not able to attend. Santa kneels next to their bed so they can have their photo taken with him as well.

*For more on what Carole does in nursing homes,
see page 60. To contact Carole, see page 190.*

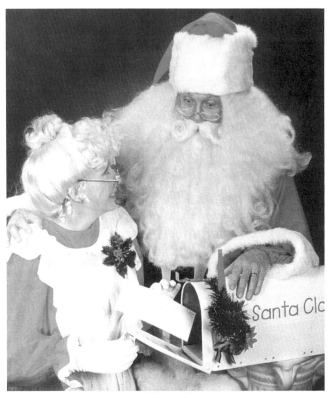
*Ruth and Tom Matteson*

## Experience the Real Magic of Christmas

By Ruth "Angell" Matteson

If you are already Santa or Mrs. Claus, you have touched many hearts and brought back memories and moments of excitement to all you have encountered. If you aren't Santa or Mrs. Claus, you haven't experienced the real magic of Christmas.

The "thank-you's" that you receive from those who cross your path are the glowing smiles, wide opened eyes, laughter and hugs. You are a magical animation, a part of their past.

My husband and I have been Mr. and Mrs. Claus since 1995. We attended Charles W. Howard Santa School for several years. That's an experience in itself. There is contact information at the end of this chapter if you are interested.

### You Can Feel the Excitement

When you enter a nursing home the room gets brighter—you can feel the excitement. The residents are so happy to see you. You are bringing back part of their childhood. They are just like

> The residents are so happy to see you. You are bringing back part of their childhood.

children, listening to every word you say. They will admit if they have been naughty, and they are proud of it. You get a warm feeling in your heart as you visit with these wonderful people.

### Precautions to Take

My Santa, Tom, removes his gloves before we enter a nursing home so the residents can feel the warmth of his hands as they sit and talk. You must take the same precautions you would visiting as a clown, such as washing your hands before and after your visit, and checking to see if they can have candy canes. It's best to give the nurses some candy canes to bring to the residents that are able to have them.

### About Gifts and Pictures

Ask ahead of time if the nursing home is going to be providing small gifts for Santa to hand out. If so, bring your Santa Bag and put the gifts in it without the residents seeing. If not, leave your bag in the car. You may be getting their hopes up about receiving a gift from Santa. The residents know that you are not really Santa or Mrs. Claus, but they love to play the game and keep your secret.

Find out if the nursing home has a camera and whether they will be taking pictures of the residents and Santa. Don't forget the staff. They love Santa too.

Tom and I work as a team. Being married to your partner makes everything run smoother. If you are a Santa working with a different Mrs. Claus, you need to coordinate with her on everything. Santa is the "Big Guy." Mrs. Claus is second in command. She makes sure everything is running smoothly. She keeps Santa informed as to what is coming next and when it's time to go, without making it obvious to the residents.

## *Making Jingle Bell Holders*

We hand out jingle bells to as many residents as we have bells and then sing "Jingle Bells" together. They love that they can participate. For the first 11 years I made the bells using one red and one green pipe cleaner and twisting them together. I then added three bells and connected the ends together to make a circle so they could hold the bells.

I get my bells from a hobby store after Christmas when they are marked down. You can find bells in the shape of a wreath or a candy cane with lots of bells on them. It's a lot less expensive buying them that way. I just cut the wire and take the bells off.

This year I changed to a metal ring with a hinge at the bottom and it opens at the top. I put spacer beads in-between three bells to give them more color. I carry the bells on a large metal ring made out of a heavy wire (actually it's the wire that the bells came on from the candy cane or wreath.) The wire is shaped into a circle with a hook curved at one end and a loop at the other end to connect it together. After we are through singing our song, we collect the bells and put them away.

If someone doesn't want to give his or her bells back, let them go. Either they will give them back later, or one of the staff will get them back for you. You are not the enforcer. You do no harm and say no harsh words.

## *Happy Headbands*

Over the years, we also have collected many different kinds of antler headbands. In the past few years we have included headbands such as Christmas trees, candy canes, angel halos, bobbing reindeers, Santa, Frosty, and many more. We have over 30 headbands. We pass these out and the residents love it.

It's a great photo opportunity for the whole group. We then sing "Rudolph the Red Nose Reindeer."

We spray our bells and headbands with a disinfectant after each visit so we are not spreading germs from one person to the next. This is especially important for nursing homes.

The nursing home will probably have a Christmas tree set up. Ask them if they can set up two chairs (sometimes they think

Mrs. Claus doesn't need to sit down) in front of the tree for pictures. You might want to let the residents leave their headbands on for their picture with Santa. Mrs. Claus will be able to collect it after their picture. Again, if they want to keep it, let it go and let the staff handle it.

Some residents don't celebrate Christmas with Santa and may leave the room or say something negative out loud. Don't let this discourage you. Everyone has his or her own beliefs and all are welcome to stay or leave. It's nothing you've said or done. Just go on with your visiting.

### Having Them Sit on Laps

The elderly love to sit on Santa's lap. You may even bring tears to their eyes. Just keep talking to them and let them know they are on the "Nice" list.

Some of the heavier residents may hesitate to sit on your lap. Reassure them that it will be all right, unless you have knee or leg problems; then have another chair for them to use. Don't insist that anyone sit on your lap.

Don't promise them anything. If they ask for something, tell them, "I'll see what I can do," or, "I'll add that to your list."

When it's time to leave, Santa stands up and rings his big bells and with a "Ho Ho Ho" we are out the door. We follow up the next day with the director of the nursing home to see how everything went in her eyes and to see if she has any tips that we could use in the future.

I hope you have as much fun and enjoyment as Santa and Mrs. Claus as Tom and I do. We wish you a magical Christmas with all your visits.

*To contact Ruth, see page 194. Also see her article in the next chapter.*

### Santa Claus School

For information on the Charles W. Howard Santa Claus School established in 1937, contact the School at 2408 Pinehurst Court, Midland, MI 48640 USA. Telephone (989) 631-0587 Website: www.santaclausschool.com

---

**"He errors who thinks Santa enters through the chimney. Santa comes through the heart." –***Charles W. Howard*

---

# Chapter 10
# Junior Joeys: Guidelines for Youth Clowning

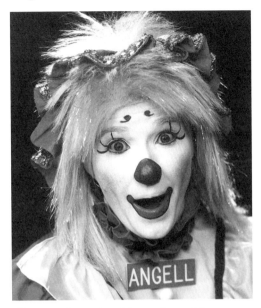

## Clowning in Nursing Homes
### By Ruth "Angell" Matteson

Junior Joeys are children between the ages of 5 and 15. Joey is another name for clowns.

### *Where Did "Joey" Come From?*

Where did the name Joey or Junior Joey come from? Between 1779 and 1837 a man named Joseph Grimaldi was the most famous and popular of all the clowns in harlequinade and pantomime. Joseph Grimaldi was the original "Clown Joey," the term "Joey" being used to describe clowns since his day.

### *You'll Need Training*

The first thing you need before going into a nursing home is training. This could be training that your clown alley provides, or one on one with an adult that has had training and has made previous visits. (Visit www.worldclownassociation.com/ and www.coai.org/ for their national Junior Joey programs.)

---

### Contacting the Nursing Home

Nursing homes have rules and regulations that you will need to abide by. Your visit will be much more successful if you know the do's and don'ts.

Contact the nursing home where you would like to visit. Find out what their policy is for you to come and do a skit, do balloons, visit with the residents, or whatever you want to do. The Director or Activity Director should be your contact person. Let him or her know what you would like to do and any training that you have completed. Find out what date and time would work for them and set up an appointment.

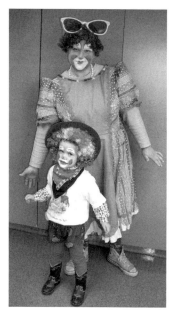

*Nursing Home residents love seeing young clowns. Above is Jodi "Ruby Doobie" Rice with her daughter Sunni a.k.a "Jo Jo."*

### Your Audience

Now you can make plans on what you are going to do to entertain the adults. Most of the time there will be children, grandchildren, staff member's children, and friends of the residents present. Each one of these people would love to interact with you.

### Ideas for Visiting and Entertaining

If you are going to be doing a skit, it's best you do that first. This will get your audience excited and used to you being in their "home." (See skits in the next chapter.)

You might want to do balloons, but don't become a balloon machine—take turns with other Junior Joeys or adults. You can visit with the residents and family members one on one. You can do magic, a walk around, or just sit and talk to them.

Some of the time the residents don't have visitors, so they are happy to talk with you. Ask them questions about their past, what was their favorite toy, what games did they play when they were your age, how many children do they have, what is their favorite holiday? If you normally wear gloves, take them off and hold their hand. They like to have human contact.

Ask the director if you could bring in your pet. Make sure your pet is well behaved around strangers and that your pet has relieved itself outdoors before entering the nursing home. The residents love to pet your animal. This is a good opportunity to talk to the resident about your pet. Ask them if they had pets when they were your age. If your pet gets too anxious, it's time for them to leave. (See tips on dog visits on page 68.)

### *Things You Should Do*

Wash your hands before you come in contact with the residents. You don't want to pass on germs. Also, wash your hands when you leave. You can use wipes, but not in front of the residents.

Show them respect, the same as you would any other adult. This is their home and you are a guest.

Try to get them involved in what you are doing—magic, walk arounds, singing, playing bingo or using them as a helper. Even if they are in wheelchairs, they can still participate as your helper when doing a magic trick. If they show signs that they don't want to participate, let them know it's all right and move on.

Include the children and their families in your antics, but focus on the residents. The staff members are also excited to see you so you should try to include them in some way.

Try to mingle with the residents. You may sit down with one of the elderly and spend some time with them, but the other residents want to interact with you also.

If it's time to leave and you are talking with one of the residents and they don't want you to go, try to make eye contact with one of the staff members to help you. They are very well skilled to handle this type of situation. If you are planning on returning, let them know you will be back to visit them.

If a resident wants to hug you and that's all right with you, go ahead and hug them. Like I said before, they love human contact. If they won't let you go, again, try to make contact with the staff for help.

## Adopt a "Grandparent"

Think about adopting one of the residents you have made contact with several times that you feel comfortable with. You could visit him or her in costume or out of costume. You will make this person feel very special.

Think of him or her as a Grandparent. Your adopted Grandparent will be very excited to see you each time you come to visit. If you can, visit them once a week or once a month.

Bring something you made especially for them. They will be sure to put it up in their room. The days are long for those living in a nursing home and your visit makes the day go by faster for them. It gives them something to think about and remember. You will be very special in their lives, especially if they don't have visitors stopping by to see them.

## Things You Should Not Do

Do not pass out candy or any kind of food unless you have received permission from the staff. You don't know if the residents are diabetic or allergic to these items.

Don't try to get them out of their wheelchair. You don't know if they can walk or not.

## Questions to Consider

After you leave, talk with your group about your experience. Did you have a good feeling about interacting with the elderly? Did you feel uncomfortable being around them? Would you like to make another visit? How often would you like to visit? Do you just want to stay at the same nursing home, or would you like to visit another one?

Consider visiting other places such as Volunteers of America Homesteads (http://www.voa.org/) which are present in 29 states. These are not nursing homes. The residents have their own apartments. An on-site nurse gives them their medication.

I hope you enjoy your visits to nursing homes and have a learning experience that stays with you throughout your life.

*Ruth Matteson is Junior Joey Director for the World Clown Association. Email Ruth at ANGELL6000@aol.com. For more on Ruth see page 194.*

**See pictures of youth clowning in Russia and China on Pages 38 and 41.**

# Kids as Clowns: Serving Through Humour

By Karen "Rootin' Tootin' Newton" Baxter

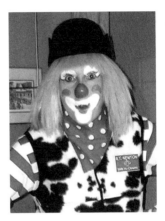

*Karen "Rootin' Tootin' Newton" Baxter*

In 2000, while working at Clover Bar Junior High, in Sherwood Park Alberta, Canada, I founded a group called KIDS AS CLOWNS. My intention was to empower youth with clowning skills so they could impact the lives of others through humour and laughter.

Over the years, approximately 140 kids have gone through the program, logging hundreds of volunteer hours and becoming "HUMOR-itarians" in our community. We "jest for the health of it" and enable people of all ages to feel hopeful and optimistic about their lives. Ten of the KIDS have even attended Clown Camp® in Wisconsin with me.

Today, KIDS AS CLOWNS regularly visits two of our local Care facilities for seniors. The KIDS visit on Saturday mornings, putting on a show for Alzheimer residents and then doing walk-arounds in the Long Term Care Unit as well as the secured Alzheimer's unit.

As part of the KIDS program and with the approval of our Board of Education, we began offering "Clowning: A Red Nose

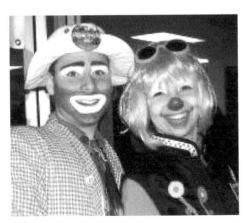

Option" to seventh grade students at Clover Bar Junior High School in the fall of 2006. I currently facilitate the program for 25 seventh graders.

*Chris "Buddy" Lewis (left), now 19, has been clowning since he was 12. He is shown with Tracy "Crazy Oopsy Daisy" Smith, a fourth grade teacher.*

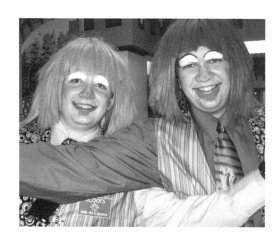

**Honored for Service**
*17 year-old twins Chris "Scoots" Fuhrmann (left) and Ryan "Sniffles" Fuhrmann who have been with KIDS AS CLOWNS since they were 12, received a "Pride of Strathcona County Award" from the Mayor for their volunteer service.*

## Another Program: HOPE KIDS

In addition to KIDS AS CLOWNS, I also visit Care Centres with youth in another program known as HOPE KIDS. HOPE KIDS are children and youth, ages 10 to 17, who are trained to share their "hope" with seniors at Care facilities through games, crafts, theme days and stories.

The program is sponsored by the HOPE FOUNDATION of Alberta which is affiliated with the University of Alberta. The Hope Kids wear regular

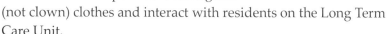

(not clown) clothes and interact with residents on the Long Term Care Unit.

I have been a HOPE KID facilitator since 1998. This year, approximately 10 Junior High students, another staff member, and I visit the seniors each week at Capital Care Strathcona. We leave school at 3:30 p.m. and visit with seniors until 5:00 p.m.

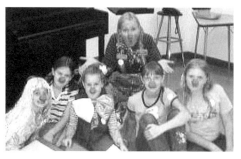

*For more details about KIDS AS CLOWNS and HOPE KIDS contact Karen Baxter at 86 Woodstock Drive, Sherwood Park Alberta Canada T8A4E2. Telephone: 1-780-464-6617 Email: karen.baxter@ ei.educ.ab.ca. or rt_newton@yahoo.ca For more about Karen, see pages 106, 138 and 188.*

# Chapter 11: Skits

*These classic skits have been performed through the years in so many variations that they are "in common usage." It is how you adapt the skit that makes it your own. For some popular skit books, see page 173.*

## Skits from Paul "Fuddi-Duddy" Kleinberger

Here are some of the skits that our alley has used in the past that play well in nursing homes and assisted living facilities.

## The King With A Terrible Temper

Props: An identification sign for each character.
       A King's crown & scepter.
       A funny hat for the Short Short Daughter.
       A different color hat for the Tall Tall Daughter.
       A fancy hat for the Beautiful Young Daughter.
       A sash or belt, scabbard and sword for the Prince.
       A broom stick horse as the Fiery Steed.

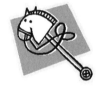

Audience Responses:

| | |
|---|---|
| King with A Terrible Temper: | **GRRRRR** |
| Short Short Daughter: | **Ohhhhhhhhhh** |
| Tall Tall Daughter: | **Whistle** |
| Beautiful Young Daughter: | **Hubba Hubba** |
| Handsome Young Prince: | **Ah Hah** |
| Fiery Steed: | **Slap Hands on Knees for Gallop** |

Narrator: "Once upon a time in a big castle there lived the King With A Terrible Temper.

Audience: **GRRRRR**

Narrator: He had three daughters: his Short Short Daughter,

Audience: **Ohhhhhhhhhh**

Narrator: his Tall Thin Daughter

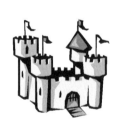

Audience: **Whistle**

Narrator: and his Beautiful Young Daughter.

Audience: **Hubba Hubba**

Narrator: In another land there lived a Handsome Young Prince

Audience: **Ah Hah**

Narrator: and his Fiery Steed.

Audience: **Knee Slapping** as a person on a horse gallops across the stage.

| | |
|---|---|
| Narrator: | One day the Handsome Young Prince |
| Audience: | **Ah Hah** |
| Narrator: | rode his Fiery Steed |
| Audience: | **Knee Slapping** as a person on a horse bounds across the stage. |
| Narrator: | up to the castle of the King With A Terrible Temper. |
| Audience: | **GRRRRR** |
| Narrator: | I have come to find myself a wife from among your daughters, said the Handsome Young Prince |
| Audience: | **Ah Hah** |
| Narrator: | to the King With A Terrible Temper. |
| Audience: | **GRRRRR** |
| Narrator: | The King With A Terrible Temper |
| Audience: | **GRRRR** |

| | |
|---|---|
| Narrator: | presented his first daughter, the Short Short Daughter. |
| Audience: | **Ohhhhhhhhhh** |
| The Prince: | No, I cannot marry her. She will eat too much, |
| Narrator: | said the Handsome Young Prince. |
| Audience: | **Ah Hah** |
| Narrator: | The King With A Terrible Temper |
| Audience: | **GRRRRR** |
| Narrator: | presented his Tall Thin Daughter. |
| Audience: | **Whistle** |
| The Prince: | No, I cannot marry her. She is too tall for me, |
| Narrator: | said the Handsome Young Prince. |
| Audience: | **Ah Hah** |
| Narrator: | Just then the Beautiful Young Daughter |
| Audience: | **Hubba Hubba** |
| Narrator: | appeared on the stairway. |
| The Prince: | I will marry your Beautiful Young Daughter, |
| Audience: | **Hubba Hubba** |
| Narrator: | said the Handsome Young Prince. |
| Audience: | **Ah Hah** |
| Narrator: | He scooped up the Beautiful Young Daughter, |
| Audience: | **Hubba Hubba** |
| Narrator: | ran out of the castle, jumped on his Fiery Steed *Continued* |

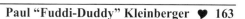

| | |
|---|---|
| Audience: | **Knee Slapping** |
| Narrator: | and rode off towards his home in a cloud of dust. As the cloud of dust settled, all that could be seen was the Handsome Young Prince |
| Audience: | **Ah Hah** |
| Narrator: | riding away with the Beautiful Young Daughter |
| Audience: | **Hubba Hubba** |
| Narrator: | on the Fiery Steed. |
| Audience: | **Knee Slapping** |
| Narrator: | So ends the story of the King With A Terrible Temper, |
| Audience: | **GRRRRR** |
| Narrator: | his Short Short Daughter, |
| Audience: | **Ohhhhhhhhhh** |
| Narrator: | his Tall Thin Daughter, |
| Audience: | **Whistle** |
| Narrator: | his Beautiful Young Daughter, |
| Audience: | **Hubba Hubba** |
| Narrator: | the Handsome Young Prince |
| Audience: | **Ah Hah** |
| Narrator: | and the Fiery Steed." |
| Audience: | **Lots of Loud Knee Slapping** |

## Adaptations

I try to find an aide who looks like fun and ask them to help. Once I couldn't find an aide so I asked a resident to hold the horse and tap it on the floor. He tried to get up and ride the thing and almost fell so now if I can't find an aide to help I do it myself. Take it slow and easy so everyone can have time to GRRRR and Ohhhhh and Ah Hah.—*Judy Barker* (see page 81)

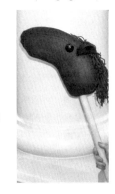

I adapted the script to use soft felt hats. The Short Short Daughter was a "real chick" (to use the Chicken Hat). The Tall Tall Daughter made the room "light up" (to use the back of the Birthday Candle Hat). I printed the signs from my computer and used a free on-line clip art growl-y face to go with the "GRRRR."

Linda "Buttons" Forrest made the "Fiery Steed" (at right) from a man's brown sock stuffed with polyester filling, buttons for the eyes, felt for the ears and yarn for the mane.—*Anita Thies*

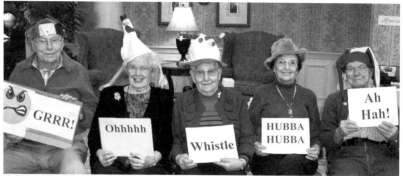

*A "tip of the hat" to these fun story leaders at Brookline, State College, PA: (from left) Bill Shoemaker, Norene Bigelow, Ruth Bittner, Helen Ciletti and Henry Hanson.*

## Taking My Case to Court

Props: A chair, an attaché or business briefcase.

A clown comes in to stage right or left. A second clown walks out on stage carrying a briefcase

First Clown: "Hey,_____, where are you going?"

Clown Two: "I am taking my case to court!"

Both Clowns: Smartly leave the stage.

First Clown: Returns to the stage.

Clown Two: Comes back out on stage carrying his/her brief case and a chair. Stops at center stage. Sets the chair down. Stands next to the chair facing the audience.

First Clown: "Hey,_____, where are you going now?"

Clown Two: Climbing on to the chair. "I am taking my case to a higher court!" Presents the case to the audience.

Both Clowns: Smartly leave the stage and remove the chair.

First Clown: Returns to the stage.

Clown Two: Comes back out on stage crying, sobbing and generally making a big fuss. He/she is carrying no props at all.

First Clown: "Hey, _____. What's the matter?"

Clown Two: Takes out a big handkerchief and blows nose loudly. "I lost my case!"

# Peanuts

Props: A desk or table, 2 chairs.

Clown Bailiff: "Hear Ye, Hear Ye, All rise. Court is now in session. The Honorable Judge ____ presiding."

Clown Judge: Comes in and sits behind the desk.

Clown Bailiff: "Thank you. You may be seated."

Clown Judge: "Bailiff, Please call the first case."

Clown Bailiff: "Call ____ the clown."

Clown Judge: "What's the charge?"

Clown Three: Sits down next to the judge and says, "Your honor, I have been charged with throwing peanuts to the elephant at the zoo."

Clown Judge: "Throwing peanuts to the elephant? Why that's the most ridiculous thing I have ever heard. Your case is dismissed. Get out of here. Call the next case."

Clown Bailiff: "Call ____ the clown."

Clown Judge: "What have you been charged with?"

Clown Four: Sits down next to the judge and says, "Your honor, I have been charged with throwing peanuts to the elephant."

Clown Judge: "Were you visiting the zoo?"

Clown Four: "Yes, Your Honor, I was, about 4 p.m. yesterday."

Clown Judge: "Another one? Why that's the craziest thing I've ever heard. What are you supposed to throw to the elephants? Your case is dismissed. Get out of here. Call the next case."

Clown Bailiff: "Call ____ the clown."

Clown Judge: "What's the charge?"

Clown Five: Sits down next to the judge and says, "Your honor, I have been charged with throwing Peanuts to the elephant."

Clown Judge: "Another one! Bailiff, make a note. We have to have a chat with the Chief of Police and Zoo Management. These charges are a waste of the court's time. Case dismissed. Get out of here. Next case."

Clown Bailiff: "Call the next clown!"

Clown Six: In a sling, limping, using a crutch, comes in and sits down in a huff.

Clown Judge: "OK, who are you and what's your story?"

Clown Six: "Your Honor, my name is Peanuts!"

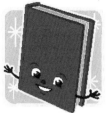

# Growing Taller

Props: A big, thick book such as a large dictionary
with a colorful cover.

A clown walks out on stage obviously engrossed in the
reading of a very large book. The book is entitled
"How to Grow Taller."

He/she walks to center stage. Faces the audience;
acknowledges them, and then keeps reading.

He/she then helps the audience understand what he/she is reading by
pointing out the title and encouraging them to repeat the title out loud.

Keeps reading. He/she suddenly puts the book down on the stage.

Steps up on the book. He/she looks around in amazement and announces,
"It works!" Takes a quick bow and runs off stage.

# The Painting

A skit for one or two clowns.

Props:  An easel, a large pad of paper, a large
paint brush and a pallet of paint.

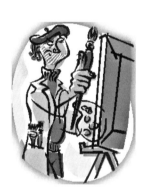

Clown:  Walks in, takes center stage and says,
"What a beautiful day to hang out in the
park! I wonder what I can do to pass
the time."

Whistles, hums, looks around.

"Wow! That is a beautiful _____.
I brought my paints with me. Maybe I will paint it."

Sets up his easel. Gets out his paints. Sticks out his thumb
to size up the _____.

"Painting is so much fun. It is so creative. Maybe when I am
finished I will take my painting over to the art museum. They put
art on display, don't you know."

Keeps painting. Puts up his thumb several more times.

"Done! Wow! This is a masterpiece!! Let me check it one more
time. What do you think?"

Shows off a picture of a large thumb, bows, then walks happily off
the stage.

# Ring Ring

| | |
|---|---|
| Props: | A long string of uninflated balloons knotted together (260s). |
| Clown One: | Enters. Takes center stage while tying balloons together in a long string. Stretching it out, he/she lets it snap back and says, "This is so cool. I have to share this with my clown friends." |
| Clown Two: | Enters the stage area. |
| Clown One: | "Hey, I have a brand new invention. It's called a telephony Would you like to see how it works?" |
| Clown Two: | "Why, yes I would." |
| Clown One: | "You take this end and go over there. Put the telephony up to your ear. I am going to say Ring Ring. You say 'Hello.' I say this is a long distance call and I have a message for ____ the clown. You say 'That's me. Give me the message.' I will let you have it (stretches the balloon and lets it snap). OK?" |
| Clown Two: | "OK." Takes one end and walks to the other side stretching out the string of balloons. |
| Clown One: | "Ring Ring.  Ring Ring.  RING RING!" |
| Clown One: | "Hey, come over here. How come you didn't say 'Hello?'" |
| Clown Two: | "I couldn't hear anything." |
| Clown One: | "You couldn't hear anything? I was practically yelling." |
| Clown Two: | "The line is all tied up." Holds up the balloon string and points to the knots. |
| Clown One: | "Come on now. That's ridiculous. Let's review. I say Ring Ring. You say 'Hello.' I say I have a message for ____ the clown. You say 'That's me. Let me have it.' I will let you have it. Do you have it?" |
| Clown Two: | "Yes, I got it." |
| Clown One: | "Go over there. Ring Ring. Ring Ring." |
| Clown Two: | Bends over and puts the balloon string up to his/her rear end. |
| Clown One: | "No! No! I said you put the telephone up to your ear, not your rear. You can't hear anything with your rear. Let's review one more time. I say Ring Ring. You say 'Hello.' I say I have a message for ____ the clown. You say 'That's me. Let me have it.' And I will let you have it." |
| Clown Two: | "OK, I have it now. Don't be mad at me. Some times it sounds like you are giving directions to a clown." |

Clown One: "Ring Ring. Ring Ring."

Clown Two: "Hello! You have reached ____ the clown's answering machine. I am so sorry but ____ the clown is not available right now. Please leave a message."

Clown One: "No, No, No. I say Ring Ring. You say 'Hello.' I say I have a message for ____ the clown. You say 'That's me, let me have it.' Let me have it! Let me Have It!"

Clown Two: "OK!" Lets the balloon string fly—*see safety caution below.*

Clown One: "Why you so and so…" Chases Clown Two off the stage in a comical manner.

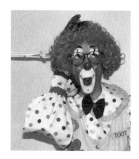

*Clown One should raise arm and elbow to protect head* **before** *Clown Two releases the balloon.*

*The head is exposed in the picture at left and is protected at right*

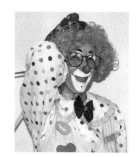

## Wrong Number

Props: Large foam telephone, a ringer.

Clown One: Enters, presents telephone and says, "When I got this phone it rang all of the time. I had lots of fun talking to all my friends. But over the last few weeks it has gotten awfully quiet."

Phone Rings.

Clown One: All excited. "Hello, is that you?"

Clown Two: Comes in stage left or right. "Of course It's me. Who is this?"

Clown One: "Sorry, wrong number."

Clown Two: "Oh, I am so sorry. I must have slipped a digit. Have a good day. Bye bye." Leaves the stage.

Clown One: "I wonder what happened. That sounded like my friend ____."

Phone Rings.

Clown One: All excited. "Hello, is that you?"

Clown Two: Steps back to previous stage position. "That's a silly question. Of course it's me. Hey, wait a minute. You sound like the last guy I talked to. Did I dial a wrong number?" *Continued*

| | |
|---|---|
| Clown One: | "You certainly did." |
| Clown Two: | "I am so sorry. I don't know what the matter is with me today. Good-bye!" Leaves the stage. |
| Phone Rings. | |
| Clown One: | "Hello, is that you?" |
| Clown Two: | Takes previous stage position. "Oh no. Wait a minute. Did I dial 555-1234? I am trying to get my friend at 555- 1234." |
| Clown One: | "Yup, you certainly did. You got 555-1234." |
| Clown Two: | "Then why do you keep telling me I have a wrong number?" |
| Clown One: | "Wrong Number? Why that's my name. I am Wrong Number." |

## Mind Reader

| | |
|---|---|
| Props: | A chair, a blind fold, a paper bag, a scarf, large plastic scissors, a pair of glasses, a wrist watch. |
| Announcer: | "Ladies and gentlemen. We are proud to have in our midst this evening ____ the clown who is just back from his/her world wind tour of ____. He/she is the greatest mind reader the world has ever seen. Please, let's welcome him/her with a great big round of applause." |
| Clown One: | "Thank you, thank you, thank you! Please, keep clapping. Thank you! Please, keep clapping. Come on now, you can clap louder and longer. Thank you. Okay now, that's probably enough. Yes, it's true. This evening we have with us ____ the clown. He/she is the world's greatest mind reader. I am his/her special assistant ____." |
| Clown Two: | Comes out on stage. Bows and takes a chair. |
| Clown One | "I am going to put this blind fold on ____. Can you see anything?" |
| Clown Two: | "What's a see?" Follows all the hand motions of Clown One. |
| Clown One: | "Maybe this isn't working. Let's try this." Puts a paper bag over the head of Clown Two. "Can you see anything now?" |
| Clown Two: | "I don't know what a see is, but I can tell you that I can't hear anything." |
| Clown One: | "Well, that just won't do." Takes off the paper bag. "Let's cover your eyes with this." Puts a scarf over their eyes. "OK, let's get started." Holds up a pair of scissors. "I am |

holding up something. Can you tell me what it is?"

Clown Two: "A bank?"

Clown One: "That's right. Give a big round of applause. Hey, wait a minute. I am not holding up a bank. Can everybody see what I am holding? Think about what this is so the great ____ can read your brain waves. ____ what am I holding? Don't run with them. Be careful when you handle them. You might cut up."

Clown Two: "I am getting an image. It's just a little fuzzy. Hold it a little higher."

Clown One: "You are sharp tonight!"

Clown Two: "You are holding a pair of scissors!"

Clown One: "That's correct. Come on ladies and gentleman. Give a big round of applause. Thank you." Holds up a pair of glasses. "What do I have now?"

Clown Two: "Please hold it a little higher so I can focus in on it."

Clown One "You should be able to see them in your mind now. Concentrate. Don't be making a spectacle of yourself. Just tell us what you see."

Clown Two: "A pair of glasses."

Clown One: "That's correct ladies and gentlemen. Give him/her another round of applause." Holds up a watch. "What do I have now?"

Clown Two: "Just a second, two, three, four."

Clown One: "Your antics are beginning to tick me off. Come on now. It's almost time for us to go. Time's a wasting."

Clown Two: "It's a watch."

Clown One: "Isn't that amazing ladies and gentlemen. Another round of applause. Well, it's time for us to leave."

Clown Two: "A tree!"

Clown One: "Come on now, we need to go."

Clown Two: "A bathroom?"

Clown One: "Stop goofing around. We have to go."

Clown Two: "A traffic light…"

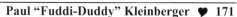

# Stage Coach

**Props:** Two chairs center stage facing the audience. A foam shot gun is placed between the chairs.

Clown One enters, takes center stage standing near a chair and says, "Boy, it looks like a great day to deliver the mail. But, I should really find somebody to ride shotgun."

Clown Two:   Enters the stage area.

Clown One:   "Howdy_____! How would like to hop the stage coach and help me deliver the mail? I will even let you ride shotgun. It's the best seat, 'ya know."

Clown Two:   "Way cool! Sounds like fun. And, it's a great day for a ride Where's the stage coach?"

Clown One:   "Why it's right here! I just have to finish hitching these fine horses to it. Climb aboard."

Clown Two:   "OK."

Clown One:   "Hey, you are in my seat. You are supposed to be in the shotgun seat."

Clown Two:   Moves over. Looks around.

Clown One:   "Buckle your seat belt. Remember, safety first."

Both clowns:   In unison, they buckle up their seat belts.

Clown One:   "Giddy up."

Both clowns:   Move like they are riding a stage coach.

Clown Two:   "So where are we taking the mail?"

Clown One:   "We are taking it over to the Central Mail Facility in Colonie."

Clown Two:   "Gee, that's a long way from here. Are there going to be any potty stops along the way?"

Clown One:   "We just left. Do you need to go potty already?"

Clown Two:   "No, no; not yet. Just thinking ahead."

Clown One:   "Ahead? When you ride shotgun, you are supposed to be looking behind."

Clown Two:   "Looking behind? What for?"

Clown One:   "Well, we're going through injun country. I don't want any of them injuns sneaking up on us. Keep your eyes open."

Clown Two:   "Injuns? You never said anything about injuns."

Clown One: "Quit your jabbering and keep a look out."

Clown Two: Looks back and says. "You better go a little faster."

Clown One: "Why?"

Clown Two: "I think there are injuns back there."

Clown One: "Giddy up. How close arc they?"

Clown Two: "I don't know, but they are this big." Indicates with fingers. Both clowns move faster.

Clown One: "How are we doing?"

Clown Two: "I don't know, but the injuns are getting closer."

Clown One: "How can you tell?"

Clown Two: "Now they are this big." Indicates with hands.

Clown One: "Giddy up. How are we doing?" Both clowns go really fast.

Clown Two: "I don't know. But, you better make those horses go faster because they are gaining on us."

Clown One: "How can you tell?"

Clown Two: "Well, now they are this big." Uses arms.

Clown One: "You better take the shot gun and shoot at them to scare them off."

Clown Two: Grabs the shotgun, aims and then stops all the action.

Clown Two: "I can't shoot at them!"

Clown One: "What do you mean you can't shoot at them? You are riding shotgun. That's your job."

Clown Two: "I have known them since they were only this big!"

## Some Skit Book Recommendations

Two of my favorites are by Barry "Bonzo" DeChant– *Anita Thies*
*The World's Funniest Clown Skits,* available from retail outlets, is 190 pages

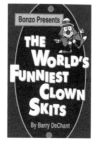
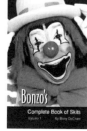

with 50 skits including popular new skits and classics with a new twist.

*Bonzo's Complete Book of Skits, Vol. 1,* is 121 pages with 39 skits from award winning clowns plus new skits and is available for $10 plus postage from Barry DeChant, 4215 64th Ave. East, Sarasota, FL 34243, bonzkari@aol.com Telephone: (941) 351-6572.

# Chapter 12: Creative Resources

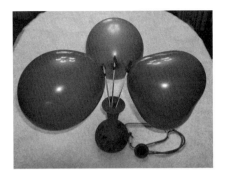

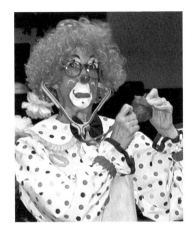

## Round Balloon Blowup
## Always Brings Laughs

This routine and the towel chicken (page 180) draw the
biggest laughs in my community room programs. You'll
want:

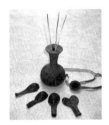

>       Three round balloons and balloon sticks
>       One 11-inch heart balloon
>       A vase so the balloons won't tip over
>       A toy stethoscope
>       Light background music such as Frank
>           Mill's *Music Box Dancer*

### Balloon One: Getting All Pumped Up

The clown fails (with loud sputtering) to blow up balloon one, then has
a "bright" idea and calls on a helper who pumps the clown's arm like a water
pump. The clown wraps the balloon onto a stick and puts it in a vase.

Your helper could be in a wheelchair. If they aren't able to reach your
elbow, extend your arm straight for them to pump your hand up and down.

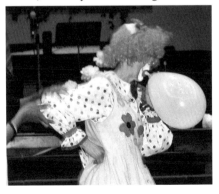

### Balloon Two:
### What an Airhead

For balloon two, hold the
balloon next to your ear while
blowing out your mouth. When
you fail at that, you have another
"bright idea" and call up a helper
to blow in your ear.

For two helpers, stand them
on either side of you to blow in

both ears. Try to find people your own height so you don't have to lean down.

Let them blow into your ears two or three times while you blow into the balloon, so the residents understand that you are an airhead. (Thanks to Bob Degen at right for helping to demonstrate.)

Then on the next blow, spit the balloon upward and out (as though the air has gone right through your head). This will draw a big laugh.

After you pick up the balloon, you mime trepidation at the power of the helpers and ask them to blow more gently.

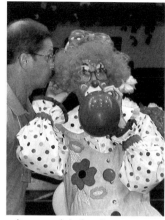

As they do, you complete balloon two and wrap it on a stick for the vase.

### *Balloons Three and Four: A New Heart*

For balloon three, signal to the residents to all "blow" at you while you blow into the balloon. This balloon needs to be red. (Balloons one and two may be any color.)

At the end, mime celebrating and "accidentally" let go of the balloon before you put it on the stick. When you retrieve it, listen to it with the toy stethoscope (see picture previous page) and mime that it has "died." Then have another "bright" idea and call on a helper. As they come up, discreetly substitute the red heart balloon and put the other balloon in your pocket.

As you hold the heart balloon, have the helper cross their hands and push down on it five times while you count and then you blow twice. They push five times. You blow twice. When the "C.P.R." is completed, you show the residents that it is a heart and everyone goes "ooohh!"

You also can add a message of three words starting with the letters C, P and R. (For a Christian version use "*C*hrist" "*P*romises" "*R*esurrection.")

# The Clown "Eye Chart" Test

I printed out each letter on 8 ½ x 11 inch colored paper and had them laminated at a copy shop. It folds in thirds for easy packing.

I present it as "the Clown Eye Chart Test with the SECRET message. We say the letters together— I Y Q. What could the SECRET message be?"

If they don't get it, you say, "I Y Q. Do you 'wike' me?" and pretend to hear the correct answer. "Yes, I LIKE you." Then distribute IYQ stickers for them to test their family and friends.

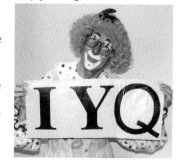

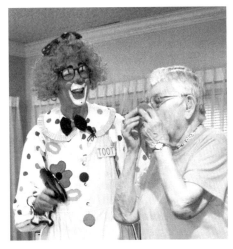
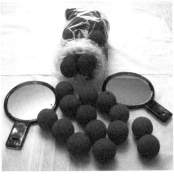

*98-year old Ruth Bittner adjusts her "new" nose during a program at The Inn at Brookline, State College, PA*

## How to Do the "Red Nose" Transplant

Supplies: Noses, hand mirrors, bubble blow, real camera.

Optional: A level, fake camera, stickers.

Foam clown noses can help residents "put on a happy face." They also can have a transforming effect when placed on family, friends, staff and administrators.

Be sure to take enough hand mirrors so they can see themselves. Take a camera to give them their picture. That way they can share the moment again and again with others.

You can do the "transplant" one-on-one or in group programs. In group situations, I like to call one to five persons upfront to demonstrate to the entire group what we are doing before noses are distributed to everyone to put on. If there's a favorite staff person who will ham it up, be sure to include them in the initial "operation."

Place your volunteers so they can be seen by the sitting group. It's best if at least one volunteer is able to stand (for visibility sake) but if they're in a wheelchair, try to create a center front aisle so others can see them.

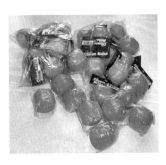

If your clown noses are individually packaged, partially open them first, cutting off the cardboard and removing any staples that held the cardboard together. Then hold onto the plastic wrapping and "push" the nose out for them to grab. There also are noses that are not individually wrapped. For links to suppliers, visit this book's website at angelfire.com/planet/nursinghomeclowning/

## How You Say It Makes It Funny

Remember that *how* you say it can be as funny as *what* you say, so have fun with your voice. I say "And now it's time for the FAAA-MOUS RED NOSE transplant. DON'T worry. It won't hurt. First I need to be sure you're on the level." (You can either hold up a big level and pretend to measure their nose—"Oh my a bubble off!"—or hold up your hands to "size" them up.)

"And for good hygiene we need to cleanse the area so I will blow a bubble for you to catch." (Or "I will provide a small bubble bath.")

**Safety alert:** Don't blow too many bubbles or get them on floors that would make residents slip. Don't get bubbles in residents' eyes. Usually I blow bubbles close to their hand so they can reach out with their fingers and then touch their nose. If you have a staff person who can "juggle" going after a bubble with their nose, the residents love that.

In offering them two noses to choose from, I say, "Notice how genteel I was—I didn't say 'pick your nose.'" Then I tell them to open up the slit in the foam nose and to place it on their nose. I hold up a mirror for them to see.

I often take a "fake" picture of the volunteer group, using a toy camera or miming with my hands. I then produce a row of smiley 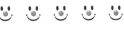 stickers that I show to the audience. (The row itself draws laughs) "Oh look, we're all related."

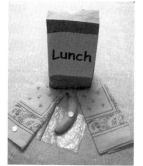

# Banana Bandana

Seniors get a kick out of the messy banana and your fun facial expressions in this popular skit.

Props: Two yellow bandanas, one banana, two quarters, brown bag with "lunch" written on it, plastic bag for your pocket.

One clown misunderstands the directions on using a *bandana* to make a quarter disappear and picks up a *banana* instead.

Because some seniors often misunderstand directions themselves, there is a softening of the message at the end.

The Scarf Clown needs to stand to the front side of the Banana Clown so he/she doesn't see the banana "mistake" in progress.

Scarf Clown:   Holding a yellow bandana and a quarter says, "I've got a new magic trick with my *bandana* where I make a quarter disappear. Would you like to see it? Oh I hope _____ the clown doesn't want to learn it because  he/she gets everything mixed up."

Banana Clown: "Hi _____ Can I learn the magic trick. Can I? Can I?"

| Scarf Clown: | "Should we let her/him?" Crowd says yes.<br>"OK. Well you need a bandana—there's one over there in my lunch bag on the table." Banana Clown takes both a banana and a yellow scarf out of the bag, looks puzzled, chooses banana and puts scarf down. |
|---|---|
| Scarf Clown: | "And you'll need a quarter " Banana Clown borrows a quarter pre-given to audience.<br>"Now first you OPEN IT UP." |
| Banana Clown: | Says, "OK" to indicate to Scarf Clown when to proceed with the next instruction. Banana clown unpeels banana, and puts peel down. Have a towel on floor to put peel on. |
| Scarf Clown: | Then improvises instructions—fold over, fold in half, left upper corner to right lower corner, etc. At one point, Banana Clown may eat part of the banana to make the banana "fold." After a few instructions, Scarf Clown says, "Then put the quarter in the middle." Banana Clown squishes quarter into the banana. "And put it in your pocket." Banana Clown hesitates to put it in their pocket. |

"Go on, put it in your pocket. And pat it three times.
One, two, three to smooth it out."
The patting can be done by either clown.

Scarf Clown has quarter shake out in his/her pocket. Banana Clown has plastic bag in pocket to protect clothes. Then Scarf Clown takes out bandana and unfolds and shows that the quarter is gone but Banana Clown says, "Mine didn't work."

| Scarf Clown: | "What is THAT? I said *bandana* not *banana*. That was my lunch." |
|---|---|
| Banana Clown: | "Here you want it?" Stretching out his hand with banana.<br>"I guess I got mixed up huh?" |
| Scarf Clown: | "Yeh but we all do sometimes. Come on, let's go get a new lunch and I'll treat us to dessert." |
| Banana Clown: | "Can we have a banana split?" |

## Chicken Cord en Blue

Say: "We had a great gourmet meal at the clown banquet—perhaps you've made it yourself." Present the chicken, the rope and the blue scarf saying with each "chicken, cord, on the color '*bleu*'" Try to give a fancy accent to the "*bleu*." Say: "Attractively arranged" as you present it feet first.

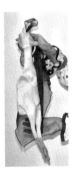

*Buckets of Love*
# What a Little "Love Dusting" Can Do
By Julie "O. B. Joyfull" Jahn

My favorite walk around in nursing homes and limited areas where seniors are plentiful is a colorful bucket with lettering all around the outside of the bucket reading "LOVE."

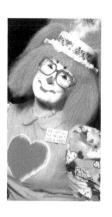

With a feather duster in hand and my "Love" bucket I go around and stimulate conversation about love. I might ask, "Did you ever hear the story about the first time I fell in love?"

Before leaving I ask them if they would like a "love dusting." The answer is usually a resounding "yes."

The seniors love it and usually open their arms wide open to receive as much love dusting as they can. When invited I always give hugs to go along with the dusting!

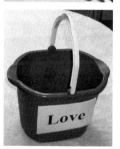

### My Favorite Experience

My favorite memory of this walk around was one time when I was in a nursing home and one resident kept watching O.B. Joyfull walk around. She was very quiet and hardly said anything.

When O.B. reached her, she said "Honey, I need more than a sprinkling of that stuff. Dump the whole bucket over me." And with that she opened her arms, stretched out her legs and gave me a big smile!

The nurse later told me she hardly every speaks or moves. WOW! It is awesome what a little bit of love dusting can do!

## The "Cat" Scan

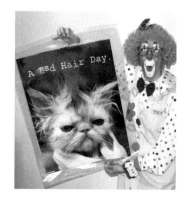

Animal pictures always bring smiles. Find one of a bedraggled cat and say it is a "cat scan" of someone who lost their sense of humor.

That's why we need our funny bone. "Have you been exercising your funny bone?" You can show a "clown" funny bone and have them point to and flex their elbow. Then tell corny jokes.

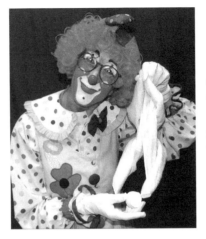

# How to Make
# the Towel Chicken

Have a volunteer hold their arms straight out and roll the towel on their arms while humming a circus-y tune.

I'll say, "Have you ever had to make something from scratch. This is what we did for our clown banquet."

And then I make the chicken. Before you finish it, have everyone say the magic word which is "CLUCK CLUCK."

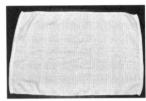
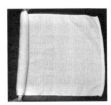
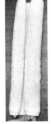
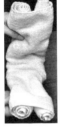

Roll each end of the towel into the middle. Fold towel back onto itself.

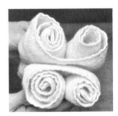
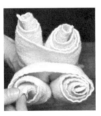
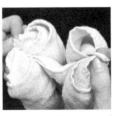

Pull out each footsie at end of towel and grip two together at each end.

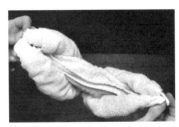
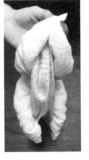
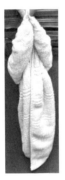

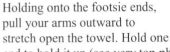

Holding onto the footsie ends, pull your arms outward to stretch open the towel. Hold one end to hold it up (see very top photo and above). For a "dressed" chicken, keep holding to top but "shake" it out at bottom.

---

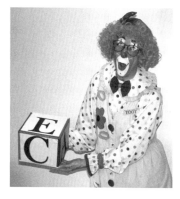

## The "Exercise Block"

Large letters printed out on colorful paper and glued to a box make a "block" for residents to walk or wheel "around the block." (I set the block on a table so they don't trip.)

I also do easy exercises by having the block go "around them." I hold it as I walk around them while they are sitting.

## Conversation Starters From Head to Toe

Accessorize your costume to bring smiles and start conversations as Peggy "Sunflower" Cole (right) does with the bird on her hat and the clamshell hanging around her neck. (She calls it her "pearl" necklace.)

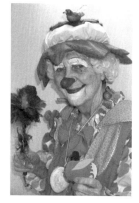

She also engages residents with her foam "apple" handouts (an "apple a day") and her bending flower prop that leads to fun talk about gardens.

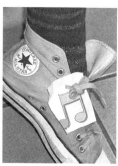

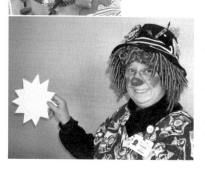

Jodi "Ruby Doobie" Rice (left) keeps out of hot water with her teabag earring.

She's only a step away from remembering song tunes with the help of her "foot notes."

Irene "MacDaddy" MacConnell-Davinroy (left) brings a little sunshine to residents with her "sun" cutouts. She uses them to affirm residents' bright smiles and also jokes about the weather. She wears a pin on her hat that says "Old Age Combat Hat and Survival Kit."

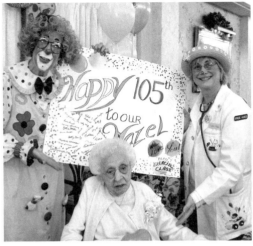
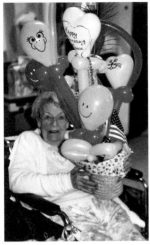

*Hazel Ryder of State College, PA celebrates her 105th birthday with me and her granddaughter Jean "DR Daisy Buttons" Lehman, a member of the Bumper "T" Caring Clowns. At right, Marie Sciullo holds a bouquet of birthday balloons created by Donna "Spangles" Shuster. This was Marie's favorite picture. Marie lived at Seneca Place, Pittsburgh. (See page 110.)*

## Making Birthdays Special

Your clowning at their birthday not only helps it to be a true celebration but lightens the load for families and staff.

Be sure to lead them in a round of the "clown birthday" song sung to the tune of "Ta Rah Rah Boom Dee Ay" with these words: *"This is Your Birthday Song; It Isn't Very Long."* Sing it with peppy clapping. After you stop singing and clapping, it will take them a moment to get the humor.

### The Magic Birthday Cake

You can make the cake with great flourish and input from the residents. You can buy "Dove" or "Chick" pans from clown dealers as well as foam birthday cakes that load into the pan lids. I say, "Let's make a cake from

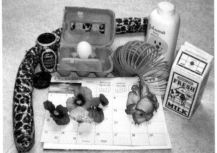

scratch. What ingredients do we need?"

Flower: Put in fresh or artificial flowers.

Egg: Be sure to put a raw egg in the pan. I ask, "Do I need the white, the yellow or the whole egg?" When they say, "Whole egg" I crack the egg and put it all in, including the shell.

Baking powder: "Oops I'm

out. Let's substitute. I'm sure you were a beautiful baby." And I hold a big bottle of baby powder above the pan and squeeze a lot out.

Sugar: "We're all watching our weight. Everybody smile and I'll put in your sweet smile."

Milk: I pour from a clown milk prop with a "cow" moo inside saying, "I stopped by a dairy so it would be fresh."

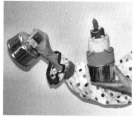

Dates: I tear off their date from a calendar.

Nuts: I use a nut jar that rattles with a small spring snake inside. I give them warning saying, "I've been having trouble with snakes getting in my pantry. Has that ever happened to you?" Be sure to release the snake back over your shoulder instead of out to them.

Then I say, "All done" but when I put my fingers into it, I pull up a gooey mess. (I take a moist towel to wipe raw egg off my hand.) "Oh, what did I forget?"

I use a rainbow slinky and say, "I forgot to put in all those good rainbow wishes for your birthday." And I move the slinky over the pan. (The slinky is too big to put in the pan.)

"Oh and we forgot to cook it. Everyone hold up your little finger and wave." (See picture above.) "It's a microwave! Let's cook it on high."(You raise your arm above your head and wave your finger up and down.)

Then say the magic word, put the lid on the pan (which releases the hidden cake) and open it up to reveal the cake. "Oh, it's a sponge cake!"

## Create Holiday Themes

Many sight gags used in parades work well in nursing homes because they can be easily seen and have a short message. Think of holiday related sight gags you could create with a clown twist. For instance, for St. Patrick's Day, I say "Have you heard the song 'When Irish Eyes are Smiling'? Do you want to see MY Irish Eyes?" And then I show them the side with the green colored "I's." (The face sign below actually has bright green I's.)

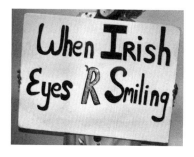

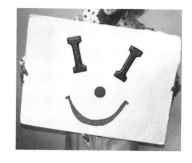

# How to Make the Napkin Rose

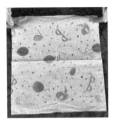 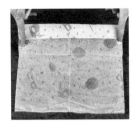 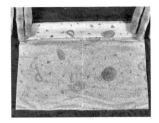

Open up the paper napkin and begin to fold it over from one end in one inch strips. Fold the same strip over and over (about 4 or 5 times) until you go just past the center fold of the napkin.

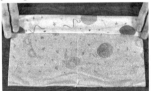 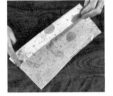 

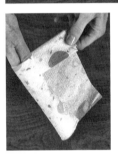 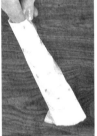 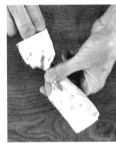 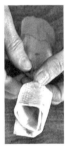

Then grip the end of the thickened part of the napkin with your two fingers (like a "scissors") and wrap the napkin around and around your fingers. When completed, remove your fingers and twist the wrapped part just beneath the thickened strip area. This will create a "cup" at the top.

Find a lose bottom outside corner of the napkin and flip it up to simulate a "leaf." Then twist beneath the "leaf" to finish the stem.

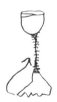 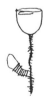 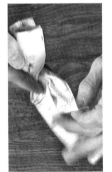 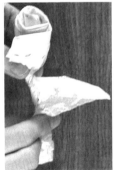

# Fly Them "Over the Rainbow"

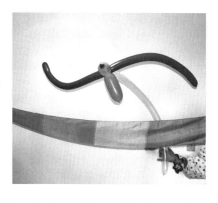

This colorful production always delights and is well worth the investment. You'll need a "change bag" (sold by clown dealers), individual small scarves, a long rainbow scarf (also sold by dealers though you might make one yourself), three balloons and a recording of "Over the Rainbow."

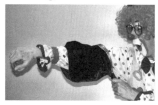

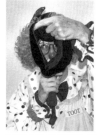

I like the change bags with zippers since you can play around first before producing the rainbow scarf. You can poke your arm through the unzipped bag or play peek-a-boo before you zip it up. You place individual scarves into the bag and then produce the rainbow scarf. Have two people hold the long scarf while you have your bird animal "bluebird of happiness" fly over the rainbow.

You can vary what you say when you put the individual scarves in the bag. Each scarf could represent a good characteristic in their life (joy, love, strength) or could represent all the different individuals in the home. The rainbow scarf brings them all together. You'll find they'll love singing along to the song.

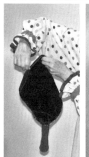
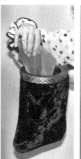
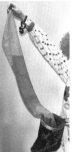

### Making the Bluebird

Balloon books from dealers can show you how to do this. Basically, you twist together an inflated "260" balloon and a "321" bee balloon. To add a handle, inflate a "260" clear balloon, twist a little bubble at one end and secure it around the neck of your bird.

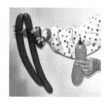
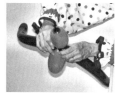
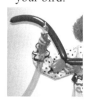

# About the Author

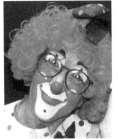

**Anita "Toot" Thies** heard God's call into clowning in the early 1980's after receiving healing from a major depression.

Anita says, "Isn't it just like God to see the potential in a depressed person and say, 'I'll heal her and make a clown of her.'" That is why her favorite scripture is "God has brought me joy and laughter: Whoever hears of this will laugh with me" (Genesis 21:6).

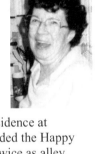

In the past 25 years, she has clowned in a variety of venues from schools and community programs to hospitals, hospice programs and churches. She has a special place in her heart for nursing homes because of the time her mom spent in one. Her mom, Ginnie Gosney, is shown on page 26 and at right in healthier days.

Anita has been privileged to teach at Clown Camp®, University of Wisconsin-LaCrosse, and at national conferences. She has co-led worship at a World Clown Association national convention and served as clown in residence at Presbyterian Women Churchwide Gatherings. She co-founded the Happy Valley Alley of the World Clown Association and served twice as alley president. She also is a member of Clowns of America International.

She is a past president and newsletter editor of Cheer Leaders for Christ and a member of its successor organization, Creative Artists for Jesus.

In 2003, she co-authored *The Joyful Journey of Hospital Clowning: Making a Difference with Love and Laughter* (Lighthearted Press).

She teaches nationally on hospital and nursing home clowning, the role of humor in health, and clown ministry.

For more, see her websites at:

www.geocities.com/toot_the_clown/ (Christian clowning)
www.angelfire.com/hi5/toot/ (Community clowning)
www.geocities.com/lightheartedpress/ (Hospital clown book)
www.angelfire.com/planet/nursinghomeclowning/ (This book)

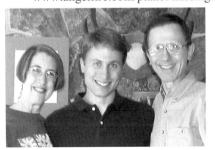

She may be reached at 761 Cornwall Rd., State College, PA 16803. Telephone: (814) 237-9466. Email: anitathies@yahoo.com

*At left Anita is shown with two laugh makers in her life—her son Bill and her husband Jim.*

# About the Illustrator

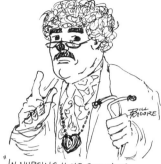

DR. MAL PRAKTISS SAYS:

"IN NURSING HOME CLOWNING, EVERYTHING IN MODERATION!"

**The Rev. Bill Moore** started drawing adventure strips for his own entertainment while in elementary school. He set his sights on becoming a professional cartoonist.

Instead, God sent him to Pittsburgh Theological Seminary where he studied to become a Minister of Word and Sacrament. Bill was ordained in 1963

After retiring in 2000, he became a "volunteer" cartoonist for a weekly newspaper. His clowning career began around 1970. His first clown character is named "Mo" from moros, a Greek word

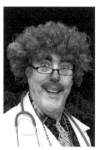

for fool, as in Fool for Christ. Lately he created "Dr. Mal Praktiss" who visits in nursing homes. Bill thanks his wife, Carol, who made Mo's clown costume and helped put together Dr. Mal's outfit.

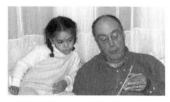

*Bill with one of the joys of his life—his granddaughter Brooke Hart.*

# About the Clown Contributors

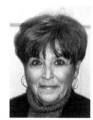

**Judy "The Cute One" Barker** (Pages 5 and 76) is founder and president of A Healthy Humor Clown Unit, Inc., that teaches clowns how to do therapeutic clowning and provides clowns to hospitals, children's facilities, hospice units, nursing homes, grief groups, assisted living facilities and Alzheimer's units.

Judy has been clowning since 1998. She received the 2002 and 2003 Clown of the Year Award from the JSH Clown Alley. Caring Clowning is her passion and she has traveled throughout the United States and Canada lecturing, teaching workshops and studying with leading professionals.

She has taught Caring Clowning at Advanced Studies in Clown Arts, at the Canadian Caring Clown Convention, at the Southeast Clown Association and at the Mid-Atlantic Clown Association. She has received training at Clown Camp® 2000 and 2001, Mooseburger Camp, and conventions of the World Clown Association (WCA) and Clowns of America International. She is the 2007 Education Director of WCA. She has written for *Funny Paper* Magazine and was featured on its cover with her infamous puppet

"Charmine." Judy clowns at Children's Cancer Clinic and Children's Hospital in Oklahoma City and organizes the "Pick Your Nose Day" fund raiser. She does in service programs for hospitals and nursing homes and works with hospice groups. She attends two summer camps for children with chronic illnesses and the state Firefighter's Burn Camp.

Contact Judy at P.O. Box 6533, Norman, Oklahoma 73070. Telephone: (405) 872-7171. Email: AHHClownUnit@aol.com

**Karen "Rootin' Tootin' Newton" Baxter** (Pages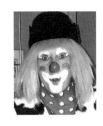
106, 138 and 160) is Education Coordinator for the
Edmonton Caring Clowns and Western Canadian Director
for the World Clown Association. She is an educator and
former pediatric registered nurse. In 2000, she founded
KIDS AS CLOWNS to empower youth to impact the lives
of others through humour. Since then, 140 kids have gone
through the program.

Karen also visits Care Centres with HOPE KIDS, youth ages 10 to 17 who are trained to share their hope with seniors. HOPE KIDS is sponsored by the HOPE FOUNDATION of Alberta. Contact Karen at 86 Woodstock Drive, Sherwood Park, Alberta, Canada T8A4E2. Telephone: (780) 464-6617. Email: karen.baxter@ei.educ.ab.ca. or rt_newton@yahoo.ca

**Brian "DR. Briny" Black** (Page 105) teaches hospital
and nursing home clowning for "The Sunshine Squad" of
the Rose City Clowns, a COAI alley in Portland Oregon.
Contact Brian at 522 N. Adair St., Cornelius, Oregon
97113. Telephone: (503) 357-9526. Email:
brinytheclown@yahoo.com

**Karen and Daniel Boudreaux** (Page 126) created FreshFire Ministries from a desire to show everyone that God loves them. "Jesus used parables to illustrate God's will for our lives. With FreshFire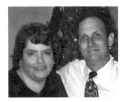
Ministries, we attempt to bring stories and songs to
life through drama, interpretive movement, dowel
rod mime, clowning and flags," say Karen and Dan.

Contact them at FreshFire Ministries, P.O. Box
839, Gray, Louisiana 70359. Telephone: (985) 872-
9576. Email: goeaglesnest@yahoo.com

**Bobbi "Kizzy" Chard** (Page 125) and her husband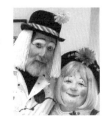
Dave "Justy Nuff" Chard do clowning, storytelling and
music in nursing homes, churches and community events.
They are members of Creative Artists for Jesus.

Contact Bobbi at 194 Norman Ave., Pleasant Gap,
PA 16823. Telephone: (814) 359-3111.
Email: bchard99@comcast.net

**The Rev. Randy Christensen** (Page 133) has taught clowning and performed in 25 states and four foreign countries. He has written more than 20 books on clowning, variety arts methods and children's ministry, a number of them translated into Spanish and Portuguese. He works full-time overseeing children's programming at a church in Willmar, Minnesota.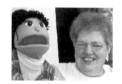

Visit his website at www.randysinfo.com/ to order his books and other resources. Visit his blog at www.pastorclown.blogspot.com/ Contact him c/o Willmar Assembly of God, 3821 Abbott Drive, Willmar, MN 56201. Telephone: (320) 235-2529. Email: pastorclown@earthlink.net

**Charlotte "Miz Frisbee" Cochran** (Page 122) and her husband Jim a.k.a."Pretzel" clown in nursing homes and hospitals. They are members of Creative Artists for Jesus. Contact them at 322 Williamson Rd., Greenville, PA 16125. Telephone: (724) 588-8284.

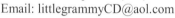

**Cathie "Periwinkle" Degen** (Page 104) clowns in hospitals, nursing homes, churches and community events. She is a member of the Bumper "T" Caring Clowns and Creative Artists for Jesus. Contact her at 2010 Hilltop Rd., Flourtown, PA 19031. Telephone: (215) 836-9332. Email: littlegrammyCD@aol.com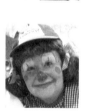

**Linda "Buttons" Forrest** (Page 27) is president of the Happy Valley Alley of the World Clown Association in State College, PA. She clowns at the Mount Nittany Medical Center in State College, at nursing homes and for a variety of community events. Contact her at 158 Presidents Drive, State College, PA 16803. Telephone: (814) 861-2605. Email: theforrests@comcast.net

**Hal "Halaloo" Grant** (Pages 121 and 131) clowns at churches, schools, festivals, fairs, birthday parties, corporate and community events and does Santa visits. He teaches clowning workshops and is a past vice president of Clowns Canada. He is a member of the Brant Alley, Brantford, Ontario, Canada and a contributor to *The Cross and the Clown.*

Hal is a member of the Fellowship of Christian Magicians, the International Brotherhood of Magicians and Creative Artists for Jesus.

"God has given me much through clowning," says Hal. "I have visited places that I never would have imagined, going to Nicaragua for instance. And I have met friends around the world. I feel blessed every time I have the opportunity to clown."    *See Hal's contact information on the next page.*

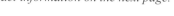

Contact Hal "Halaloo" Grant at 2473 Shurie Road, Smithville, Ontario, Canada LOR2AO. Telephone: (905) 957-0661. Website: www.Halaloo.com Email: halalootheclown@sympatico.ca or halaloo@halaloo.com

**Julie "O.B. Joyfull" Jahn**, L.L.C., (Pages 5, 114 and 179) is a nationally known clown, educator, and Christian conference leader. She is a past president of the World Clown Association (WCA) and has received awards from the WCA and the Sacred Heart Institute for her service and devotion.

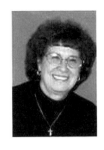

She is the founder and a past president of Cheer Leaders for Christ, an organization that equipped and nurtured those in creative ministry from 1991 through 2006. She is a member of Creative Artists for Jesus.

She has been an executive administrator and event coordinator in the corporate world for more than 30 years and a professional clown for more than 20 years. She has performed and taught in Canada and Europe as well as throughout the United States. She has lectured at many international clown conferences and has conducted several "spirituality workshops" in the U.S. She is the author of several Creative Ministry booklets and produced a Christian children's video, "Jesus Loves You."

Today Julie leads conferences, workshops and retreats focusing on changing your life through laughter, joy and creative ministry. Her topics include Landscaping a New Life, The Power of a Joyful Heart, Introduction to Creative Ministry, and My Life in a Box, in which she gives her personal testimony using a box of ordinary objects and humor. Julie says her mission is "to demonstrate through Creative Ministry the joy, laughter and love that our Lord Jesus Christ has for each one of us."

Contact Julie at 206 Clearbrook Road, Matthews, North Carolina 28105-5706. Cell phone: (704) 560-9202. Email: urblessed@carolina.rr.com Website: www.angelfire.com/planet/julieajahn

**Carole "Pookie" Johnson** (Pages 5, 60 and 150)
After becoming a clown in 1990, Carole found her specialty and passion in hospital and nursing home clowning. She clowns weekly at Children's Hospital and Regional Medical Center in Seattle and Stevens Hospital in Edmonds, WA as well as nursing homes in her area. She also is involved in pet visits.

Carole believes in the therapeutic benefits of humor and laughter, and she is proof that the blessings work both ways for the receiver and the giver. It is her dream that there be a clown in every hospital. To help her dream come true she has taught classes on Caring Clowning at Clown Camp®, University of Wisconsin-LaCrosse, and at clown conferences in the U.S., Canada, England and Japan.

Contact Carole at 1602 Locust Way, Lynnwood, WA 98036-9017. Telephone: (425) 481-7143. Email: clownjuglr@aol.com Her husband Bruce "Charlie" Johnson has books and clown resources at his website: www.charliethejugglingclown.com

**Carol "Blossom" Kay** (Pages 5, 96 and 131) is a full time professional clown and family entertainer who also operates her own bed and breakfast.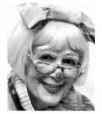

A clown since 1982, she does comedy magic, storytelling, balloon sculpting, flannel graphs, face painting, skits and gives her Christian testimony. She performs at company openings, birthday parties, picnics, Christmas parties, day cares, schools, hospitals, and nursing homes. Her main clowning is done in churches, and she has done clown ministry in schools and churches in the West Indies.

She is a member of the Toronto Clown Alley, The Fellowship of Christian Magicians, Simcoe Clown Alley and Creative Artists for Jesus. She has taught at many clown conferences. She was named female clown of the year at the PONY Convention in Erie, PA. Her motto is "to bloom where I am planted" and she says, "I have been enjoying God's 'Son' all my life."

Contact Carol at 33 Mulock Drive, Box 363, Bradford, Ontario, Canada L3Z2A9. Telephone: (905) 775-0088. Toll-free Canada 1-888-627-6690. Email: blossomb-b@on.aibn.com Websites: www.blossomtheclownbandb.com and www.bbcanada.com

**Jan "Jaepers" Kerr** (Page 120) is "Head Fool" of the Merrimakers Clown Ministry of the Aldersgate United Methodist Church in Wilmington, Delaware. Merrimakers is an interdenominational, Bible-based, Spirit-led troupe for seasoned and new clowns. Members clown in hospitals, nursing homes, care facilities, schools, festivals, churches and community events.

"Clowning is a gift from God which enables us to connect with neglected and lost persons in our community," says Jan. "It provides a way to minister to those who suffer physically and emotionally. There also is a strong presence of the clown in children's faith activities and in schools."

Contact Jan at 695 Burdett Drive, Hidden Valley, Aston, PA 19014. Telephone: (610) 485-7546. Email: merrimakers@comcast.net or jaepersclown@comcast.net

---

 **To Connect with Clowns Everywhere**

Clowns of America International  www.coai.org and World Clown Association worldclownassociation.com

---

**Paul "Fuddi-Duddy" Kleinberger** (Pages 5, 43 and 162) is internationally known for his clowning, teaching and leadership as president of Clowns of America International (COAI) and as co-founder of Red Nose Response, Inc., that mobilizes trained clowns to respond to disaster situations.

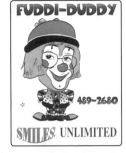

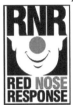
Through his Smiles Unlimited L.L.C., he clowns hundreds of times each year in all venues. He performs as "Fuddi-Duddy," a laughable klutz; the "Fantastical Mr. Fuddi," the mischievous twin brother of "Fuddi-Duddy" and "Dr. Jest Kidding," a caring clown specializing in ailments of the funny bone. He is active in numerous alleys and clown arts organizations. Outside of clowning, he has had a varied career in family entertainment, government service, law enforcement, logistics and transportation, and sales and marketing.

Contact him at 2 Maple Lane North, Loudonville, NY 12211. Telephone: (518) 489-2680. Email: fuddiduddy@aol.com Website for COAI: www.coai.org/ For Red Nose Response: www.rednoseresponse.org/

**Susan "Pancakes" Kleinwachter** (Pages 5 and 86) known as the "Queen of Theme" hails from the Chicago area. She is an entertainer who wears many hats. Her passion is laughter and humor with people of all ages. She is an award-winning clown, storyteller, teacher and public speaker who has presented in Canada, Mexico, the United Kingdom and across the U.S. including Alaska.

She customizes themes and education into her entertainment which totals hundreds of events each year including those in nursing homes, corporate events, family gatherings, fairs, festivals and more. She also performs in many different characters and incorporates music, magic, miming, balloon twisting, face painting, games, storytelling, audience participation and some good old fashion "FUN."

Susan has written several books on entertaining and has several more in the works involving the art of storytelling and some unique children's books. In 2002, she joined with Jose and Alicia Elizondo to create "Projecto Risa" (Happy/Healthy Living) which offers workshops in Monterrey, Mexico on health and humor and becoming a caring clown. Their company bought the rights to translate *The Joyful Journey of Hospital Clowning* into Spanish. This book is the first of its kind in Spanish to help with the understanding of what health and humor is all about and how it is applied in hospitals.

Susan is a member of the World Clown Association, Clowns of America International, Northern Clown Association, Chicago Guild, West

Suburban Clown Troupe, Texas Clown Association and AATH —Association For Applied and Therapeutic Humor. Susan's company, "KleinTime Entertainment," sells many products including "free B's", unique hats and headbands, paper hat tear magic tricks, zany sayings for badges and personalized badges—Example: Humor Therapist, I Suffer from Humoroids —games for people with sensory impairments, music for nursing home entertainment, books and much more. Contact Susan at P.O. Box 700, Warrenville, Il. 60555. Telephone: (630) 393-7714 (work) (630) 464-3863 (cell). Email: KleinTime @sbcglobal.net  Website: www.KleinTime.com

**Aurora "BeBop" Krause** (Pages 5 and 91) is from San Antonio, Texas. She has been clowning for the past 11 years. Her clown character "BeBop" works with children and adults in hospitals, nursing homes and hospice settings as well as charity events, parades, festivals and parties. She enjoys performing musical skits and comedy routines for audiences of all ages.

Aurora has won top honors in various categories of make-up/costume and single and group skit competitions at state, national and world conventions. In 2002 she received the "All Around Clown" award from the World Clown Association (WCA) and is currently serving on the WCA Board as Southwest Regional Director. She has served on the Texas Clown Association (TCA) Board and is currently the Education Director for TCA. In 2006 Aurora was awarded the highest award given to a Texas Clown—the "2006 Ambassador of Clowning" Award.

She has taught clowning at a local school district for the past five years and served as instructor at various clown conventions such as WCA in 2004 and 2007, Joey to the World in 2006 and 2007 and Clown Camp®, University of Wisconsin-Lacrosse in 2005, 2006 and 2007.

In her world away from clowning, Aurora has been a banker for the past 31 years and is currently a Senior Vice President in operations and management for a local bank. She lives in San Antonio with her very supportive husband Don and a spoiled german shepherd named Nelson.

Contact Aurora at 661 Richfield Dr., San Antonio, TX 78239-2011. Telephone: (210) 656-3057. Email: bebopclown@hotmail.com

**Luella Krieger** (Page 129) is a Biblical storyteller and clown. Through her ministry, Visitors from the Past, she shares the Good News of Jesus Christ through portrayals of characters from the Old and New Testaments, historic Christians and fictional characters. She and her husband Jim minister throughout the country. They are members of the National Association of United Methodist Evangelists, the Fellowship of Christian Magicians and Creative Artists for Jesus. Contact her at P.O. Box 121, Sykesville, PA 15865. Telephone: (814) 590-1937. Email: luellakk@yahoo.com Website: www.fool4christ.org/

**Jacki Kwan**, LCSW-C, (Page 18) is a speaker, workshop presenter, author, humor consultant and therapeutic clown who has been a clinical social worker since 1989. She has consulted with nursing homes, hospitals, health care providers and other organizations that deal with specific illnesses.

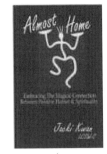

She created HA!HA!LOGY®, a multi-faceted therapeutic humor program for health care facilities. She has trained at Clown Camp® and completed Laughter Club Leadership Training. She served as a therapeutic clown on a trip to China with Patch Adams. She is a member of the National Association of Social Workers and treasurer of AATH—the Association for Applied and Therapeutic Humor. She is the author of *Almost Home: Embracing the Magical Connection Between Positive Humor & Spirituality* (2002). Jacki has become a specialist in the use of humor with Alzheimer's patients as well as those who are actively dying. Contact Jacki at P.O. Box 30769, Bethesda, Maryland 20824. Telephone: (301) 907-4610. Email: jacki@hahalogy.com Website: www.hahalogy.com/

**Ruth "Angell" Matteson** (Pages 5, 152 and 156) is an award winning clown who has taught and clowned internationally and is especially known for her work with Junior Joeys. She was a U.S. Delegate at the World Clown Congress in 1993 in Sweden and was inducted into the Midwest Clown Hall of Fame in 1996. In 2005 she received the World Clown Association's President's Humanitarian Award, only the second one to be awarded since its inception. In 2006, she was named the World Clown Association's Clown of the Year.

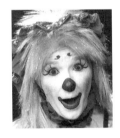

She created and established the Junior Joey educational program for the Midwest Clown Association from 1999 through 2003 and for the World Clown Association from 2001 through today. In 2002 she created and serves as editor of the International Junior Joey Cyberspace Alley Newsletter put out monthly on the Internet. She has worked with Dr. Richard Snowberg to provide a Junior Joey Camp in conjunction with Clown Camp® in 2007.

She has actively performed as Mrs. Claus since 1995 with her husband Tom as Santa. They average more than 60 visits each year which includes charity work. She is a graduate of Santa & Mrs. Claus School in Michigan where she earned her Bachelor of Santa Degree. She has served as President of Minnesota Clown Alley 19 and as President of Comedy Caravan. She has taught at numerous clown training venues including Clown Camp®, Mooseburger Clown Arts Camp and conventions of the World Clown Association and Clowns of America International.

Contact Ruth at 2764 171st Ave NW, Andover, MN 55304. Telephone: (763) 753-1593. Email: ANGELL6000@aol.com

**Tammy "Hugz" Miller** (Pages 5, 14 and 102) is the owner of Hugz and Company Consulting offering presentations on a variety of topics relating to presentation skills and coaching, humor and healing, motivation, goal setting and master of ceremony type needs. She is a motivational speaker, humorist and speech coach and holds an M.A. degree from Penn State University.

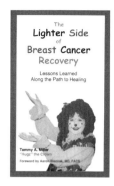

Tammy is the author of *The Lighter Side of Breast Cancer Recovery: Lessons Learned Along the Path to Healing* and the co-author of *The Joyful Journey of Hospital Clowning: Making a Difference with Love and Laughter*. She is co-founder and a past officer of The Happy Valley Alley of the World Clown Association. In 2002, she was an invited speaker at the International House of Humor in Bulgaria.

She is a Distinguished Toastmaster, currently serving as an International Director for Toastmasters International. She also is involved with Rotary International and was a nominee for the Best 50 Business Women in Pennsylvania. Call Tammy at (814) 360-4031 Email: tammy@tammyspeaks.com Website: www.tammyspeaks.com

**Pam "Sparky" Moody** (Page 118) is nationally known for L.A.F.S. (Life and Fire Safety) for Life, a non-profit organization which presents 300 safety and self-esteem assemblies annually in schools, libraries, fairs, festivals and churches.

She is Past President of the Korn Patch Klowns in Des Moines, Iowa and directs a ministry troupe, ACTS Clowns. She does clown ministry at church services, camps, praise rallies and community events.

As a caring clown, she visits hospitals, nursing homes and hospice facilities. She has taught at many national conferences including Clown Camp®, University of Wisconsin-La Crosse; Show Me Clowns for Jesus National Conference; Circus Magic; Kentucky Clown Derby; specialized Fire Inspectors' Conferences and the S.M.I.L.E. (Safety Magic In Law Enforcement) Conference. Contact her at 3108 Brookview Dr., Des Moines, Iowa, 50317. Telephone: (515) 299-3473. Email: sparky@lafsforlife.org Website: www.lafsforlife.org/

**Karen "Tickitty Boo" Oke** (Page 130) is an Office Administrator for St. Andrew's Presbyterian Church in Whitby, Ontario, Canada who is involved in a variety of ministries in her church and community. She is newsletter editor for the Toronto Clown Alley. Her clown, Tickitty Boo, is gentle but clumsy and has lots of questions about the Bible, Jesus and Heaven. The audience always seem to know how to help her (and others) figure out that God loves each and every one of us! The saying "tickety boo" means that everything is all right—and it surely is, she says, when we realize that God is in control! Contact her at gospelclown@gmail.com Telephone: (905) 430-3879. Visit their church website: www.worship-with-us.org

## Curt and Diana

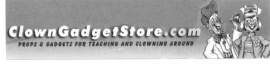

**Patty** (Page 100) travel nationally teaching and doing programs as "Handy Andy" and "Blossom." and "Doc ICU" and "Nurse Sniggles." They use clowning, puppetry and illusions to teach and entertain children and adults of all ages. As "Doc ICU" and "Nurse Sniggles," they teach caring clown skills and work in a hospital one to three days each week.

Their Clown Gadget Store offers easy to clean caring clown props appropriate for use in nursing homes and hospitals. They started clowning in 1991and today clown in churches, schools, hospitals, nursing homes and community settings. Contact them at 9335 Berry Ave., St. Louis, MO 63144. Telephone: (314) 853-5912. Email: clowngadgetstore@juno.com or handyandy.blossom@juno.com Website: www.clowngadgetstore.com

**Kathy "Popcorn" Piatt** (Pages 5 and 24) has been clowning for more than 20 years. Born in Edmonton, Alberta, Canada, she was introduced to the art of clowning by her father, Bud "Buddy" Salloum, at an early age and has been thankful ever since. She has studied in Canada and abroad, receiving a marketing degree from the University of Alberta, Sophia University in Tokyo and Penn State University. She is co-founder and past president of the Happy Valley Alley of the World Clown Association in State College, PA where she lives with her children Sean and Tavrie. She is co-author of *The Joyful Journey of Hospital Clowning: Making a Difference with Love and Laughter*.

Contact her at 195 Wiltree Court, State College, PA 16801. Telephone: (814) 235-1830. Email: kathypiatt@adelphia.net

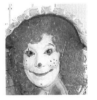

**Bud "Buddy" Salloum** (Page 25) is co-founder of the Edmonton Canada Caring Clowns that provides services to hospitals and treatment and care facilities in the greater Edmonton area. He began clowning with the Shrine Clowns in 1976 and started going to Clown Camps® in 1982. He later felt honored to be asked to instruct at Clown Camp®. He and George McEwan thought up the "Clown Camp on the Road" idea and were proud that the "masters" came to Edmonton in 1991. He and his wife Laverna live in Edmonton and are the proud grandparents of "four perfect children" (that phrase written by Buddy's son and daughter.) Contact him at 12407-135 Street, Edmonton, Alberta, Canada T5LIX8. Telephone: (780) 455-6049.

**Shobhana "Shobi Dobi" Schwebke**, M.A., (Pages 5 and 28) is a world renowned caring clown, author, teacher and artist. She is the writer, editor and publisher of *The Hospital Clown Newsletter*, an international newsletter for clowns in community and world service published since 1995.

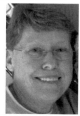

She is the co-author of *The Hospital Clown—A Closer Look: What Hospitals Need to Know About Clowns and What Clowns Need to Know About Hospitals.* She also has published a hospital clown book in Japanese.

She has worked as a hospital clown at Kaiser Permenante in Oakland, California and has taught hospital clown workshops internationally including in Japan, Portugal, England, Holland, Denmark and throughout the United States and Canada.

She has served as a clown ambassador, clowning at hospitals, schools, orphanages and historic sites on trips to Guadalajara, Mexico; Moscow and St. Petersburg, Russia; mainland China; Guatemala; and Ganeshpuri, India.

She has participated in International Cultural Festivals in England, Denmark, the Portuguese Azores, and Fukuoka, Japan. Her specialty is contemporary commedia mask character interpretation, face painting and silk magic. She has studied in Italy on a Fulbright Scholarship and holds a Master's Degree in Fine Arts from the University of California at Berkeley.

"It seems all of my experiences and life challenges were preparing me to become a clown," she says, "from my early stage experience as a dancer, through exhibiting in art galleries in New York City, to working for the New York State Division of Youth and other community services. It was as an art therapist that I learned the value of art as a medium of therapeutic communication. After moving to California, I took a clown workshop. Five minutes into my first class, my inner child popped out and refused to go back—'Shobi Dobi' was born."

"One day Shobi visited a friend in a local hospital and ended up clowning all day in the hospital's intensive care units. It was a life-changing experience and the therapeutic clown became my life's passion." Contact her at P.O. Box 8957, Emeryville, CA 94662. Telephone: (510) 420-1511. Email: shobidobi@hospitalclown.com Website: www.hospitalclown.com

**Donna "Spangles" Shuster** (Pages 5 and 108) is President of Creative Artists for Jesus, a group of Christian performing artists from the United States and Canada who serve Jesus by sharing their gifts and blessings. Members include Christian clowns, mimes, puppeteers, drama and storytellers, face painters, balloon artists and more.

Members of Creative Artists for Jesus nurture, pray for and network with one another through a free E-group and connect annually at a retreat.

Donna clowns in churches, nursing homes, birthday parties, schools and for community events. She incorporates music, illusion, drama, mime interpretations to songs, and games in her programs. She is Vice President of the Tri-Rivers Clowns in Pittsburgh, an alley of Clowns of America International. She has taught at national Christian clown conferences.

Contact her at 238 Red Oak Drive, Pittsburgh, PA 15239. Telephone: (412) 793-3902. Email: spangles2u@aol.com

**Dr. Richard "Snowflake" Snowberg** (Pages 5 and 54) is a professional entertainer, educator and Founder and Director of Clown Camp,® University of Wisconsin-La-Crosse, the world's largest and oldest clown training program. He has twice served as president of the World Clown Association. He has:

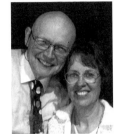

With his wife Jan

- Written five books on clowning.
- Published more than 100 articles on the art of clowning.
- Been inducted into the International Clown Hall of Fame, in 2001.
- Entertained in more than a dozen U.S. states as well as Puerto Rico, Canada, New Zealand, Scotland, England, Japan, Malaysia, Singapore and Sweden.

Richard's current clown character, "Snowflake Junior," is a goofy Auguste clown that continually gets into mischief as he tries to understand the complexities of the world around him. He has performed all over the world and is seen at corporate events, conferences, hospitals, schools, and at local festivals and fairs. His entertainment skills incorporate physical comedy, magic, storytelling, and balloons.

He developed an expertise in doing caring clown work and has also written the foremost book on the subject, *The Caring Clowns: How Humor, Smiles and Laughter Overcome Pain; Suffering and Loneliness.* He established the caring clown program at Children's Hospital of Wisconsin and has worked with many hospitals interested in incorporating therapeutic humor into their facilities.

Richard has a doctorate degree from Indiana University where he majored in Instructional Technology. He is an emeritus faculty member at the University of Wisconsin-La Crosse, where he taught in the School of Education and worked as an administrator for 27 years.

University of Wisconsin-La Crosse

CLOWN CAMP

For further information contact Richard Snowberg, 1223 South 28th Street, La Crosse, WI 54601. Telephone: (608) 796-1546 (home) (608) 785-8053 (office). Email: snowerg.rich@uwlax.edu

**Trudy "Birdie" Stryker** (Page 104) enjoys clowning at
her church, block parties, nursing homes and in parades with
the active "Goof Troupe Clowns." Contact her at 560 Zinck
Road, Jersey Shore, PA, 17740. Telephone: (570) 398-4297.
Email: cl.birdie@yahoo.com

**Korey Thompson** (Page 140) has a degree in psychology and religion and
has been clowning since 1973 in a variety of interesting places including
eldercare facilities, hospitals, colleges, conventions, cathedrals
and retreat centers. She has taught clowning at Clown Camp®,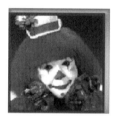
University of Wisconsin-LaCrosse, and several universities
and served for five years as architect and Artistic Director of
the Clowns for Children's Hospital of Wisconsin, Milwaukee.
    Korey is an international presenter of programs to health
care workers and teachers about relating to persons with dementia. She has
produced two videos on clowning with dementia residents. (See page 148.)
Korey currently is completing a doctoral degree in Natural Health. For her
updated postal and email addresses visit our website. (See page 200.)

**Janet "Jelly Bean" Tucker** (Pages 5 and 70) is
internationally known for her performing, teaching
and clown ministry. In 1977, she was doing marionette
shows with her husband Larry when she took a clown
class and "Jelly Bean" was born. In 1980 she began
clowning full time and performs more than 250 shows
each year for parties, picnics, corporate events,
schools, and clown ministry programs.
    She was the president of the World Clown Association (WCA) in
1990-91 when WCA had its first international convention in Bognor Regis,
England with Clowns International. She has taught clown arts at Clown
Camp®, University of Wisconsin-LaCrosse, since 1983 and taught and
performed for numerous conferences for Clowns of America International
(COAI), WCA and the Fellowship of Christian Magicians. She was an Artist
in Residence for COAI in 2002-2003.
    She was a delegate to the International Clown Summit in Dalkeith,
Scotland and has served on the Board of Directors of the International Clown
Hall of Fame in Milwaukee. She was the World Clown Association Clown
of the Year in 2002 and received the Lifetime Achievement Award of the
Midwest Clown Association in 2004. She clowned at the International
World's Fair Exposition in Aichi, Japan in 2005.
    She has written several books on clown ministry including *Skits, Bits
and Gospel Goodies; Creating Clown Stuff for Ministry; and Basic Gospel
Messages with Balloons.* You may order her books for $10 each plus
postage. Contact Janet at 6334 New Hampshire, Hammond, Indiana 46323.
Telephone: (219) 844-2858. Email: jb@jellybean-clown.com
Website: www.jellybean-clown.com/

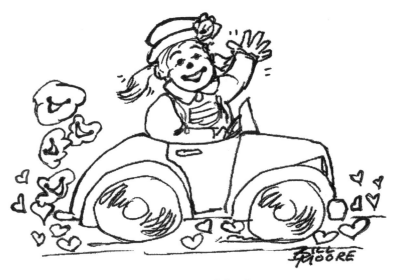

## Journey with Joy

"May we each be a clown vehicle, fueled by love, giving off
joy for exhaust, and driving on a highway of compassion."

*Shobi Dobi*

Wishing you much joy and laughter on your journey. Please
visit our website for links to clown suppliers and resources.

*Anita Thies*

**www.angelfire.com/planet/nursinghomeclowning/**

---

**For More Copies of This Book:**

An order form is on the website at:
www.angelfire.com/planet/nursinghomeclowning/

Or contact Anita Thies, Lighthearted Press
761 Cornwall Rd., State College, PA 16803
Email: anitathies@yahoo.com
Call Anita at (814) 237-9466 (home)

---